The DeFlame Diet

to

Stop your Joints, Muscles, and Bones from Rotting

By David R. Seaman, DC, MS

Author of
The DeFlame Diet
Weight Loss Secrets You Need To Know
The DeFlame Diet for Breast Health & Cancer Prevention

www.deflame.com

D1726893

Shadow Panther Press

Wilmington, NC

Disclaimer

This book is intended as an educational volume only; not as a medical or treatment manual. The information contained herein is not intended to take the place of professional medical care; it is not to be used for diagnosing or treating disease; it is not intended to dictate what constitutes reasonable, appropriate or best care for any given health issue; nor is it intended to be used as a substitute for any treatment that may have been prescribed by your doctor. If you have questions regarding a medical condition, always seek the advice of your physician or other qualified health professional.

The reader assumes all responsibility and risk for the use of the information in this book. Under no circumstances shall the author be held liable for any damage resulting directly or indirectly from the information contained herein.

Reference to any products, services, internet links to third parties or other information by trade name, trademark, suppliers, or otherwise does not constitute or imply its endorsement, sponsorship, or recommendation by the author.

Publisher: Shadow Panther Press
Cover design: www.100covers.com

ISBN: 1676029966
ISBN-13: 978-1676029960

Table of Contents

About the Author

I have been studying the relationship between diet, chronic inflammation, and pain since 1987. Below are five scientific papers I have written on this topic, which form the foundation upon which my several layperson books have been written including this one about biological rotting:

Seaman DR, Cleveland C. Spinal pain syndromes: nociceptive, neuropathic, and psychologic mechanisms. J Manip Physio Ther. 1999; 22:458-72.

Seaman DR. The diet-induced proinflammatory state: a cause of chronic pain and other degenerative diseases? J Manipulative Physiol Ther. 2002;25:168-79.

Bove GM, Seaman DR. Subclassification of radicular pain using neurophysiology and embryology. Proceedings of the 7th Interdisciplinary World Congress on Low Back & Pelvic Pain. November 9-12, 2010. Los Angeles. P.155-159.

Seaman DR. Body mass index and musculoskeletal pain: is there a connection? Chiropractic Man Ther. 2013;21:15.

Seaman DR. Weight gain as a consequence of living a modern lifestyle: a discussion of barriers to effective weight control and how to overcome them. J Chiro Humanities. 2013;20(1):27-35.

These scientific papers have been cited by researchers at Harvard Medical School on three occasions, as well as by many researchers at other universities in America, Canada, Brazil, Europe, Russia, Middle East, Africa, India, China, and Australia.

You can follow me at www.DeFlame.com, as well as at DeFlame Nutrition on YouTube and Facebook, and @DeFlameDoc on Twitter.

Introduction
Chronic inflammation and our rotting bodies

The topic of inflammation has become very popular in recent years, which is good from one perspective, but very bad from another. The problem is that "inflammation" has become a trivialized word and concept, the outcome of which is that there are many books and YouTube videos that discuss inflammation in a fashion that does not accurately characterize the issue. There are three varieties of inflammation to understand, those being acute macrotrauma-induced inflammation, low-grade microtrauma-induced inflammation, and lifestyle stressor-induced chronic low-grade inflammation.

Acute macrotrauma-induced inflammation occurs after an obvious injury, such as an ankle sprain or bee sting. It is characterized by redness, heat, swelling, and pain. This acute response typically resolves rapidly so healing can occur and there usually are no chronic effects unless the trauma was substantial.

Microtrauma-induced inflammation is not associated with redness, heat, and swelling. It is associated with pains in musculoskeletal tissues (muscles, joints, tendons, etc.), which are caused by sitting in poor posture, working for hours in constrained postures, and repetitive movements in the workplace. This type of inflammation and related pain typically resolves by avoiding the microtrauma-related activity and by getting appropriate treatments offered by chiropractors, physical therapists, massage therapists, and acupuncturists.

Chronic low-grade inflammation is very different in appearance; it is never associated with an obvious injury and there is no redness, heat, or swelling. The causes of chronic low-grade inflammation involve various lifestyle stressors, such as a pro-inflammatory diet, a lack of sleep, poor personal psychological/emotional management, sedentary living, cigarette smoking, and excess alcohol intake. The inflammation caused by these stressors is low-grade, which means there is not enough inflammation to create redness, swelling, or heat. Chronic inflammation is best viewed as a biological "rotting" process. If you view chronic inflammation in any other way, you will not properly capture its nature, as you will see in the remainder of this book. So, whenever you see the terms "chronic inflammation" or "chronic low-grade inflammation," you should be thinking, depending on the chapter, "rotting blood vessels, muscles, joints, tendons, spinal discs, and bones."

When macrotraumas and microtraumas occur in chronically inflamed people

The people who heal properly from pains caused by macro or microtrauma-induced inflammation are typically healthy to varying degrees and not compromised by the rot of chronic inflammation. In contrast, individuals who are rotting with chronic inflammation tend to not heal and develop chronic pain. These people typically do not respond to drugs, surgery, nutritional supplements, or the conservative care offered by chiropractors and physical therapists. These people need to "DeFlame" or "de-rot" their bodies. Consider the following example.

If your house was rotting, you would be concerned and get it fixed
Several years ago, I bought a house about two years before I resigned from my job. This meant I would go there on weekends and holidays, with the plan of moving in full time at some point in the future. It turned out that I had a leak in one of my windows, but I did not know it until I moved in because when I was there on weekends, it never rained enough for me to notice. Within the first year of moving in, the leak became apparent. In short, I had to open up the wall and replace the rotting wall beams.

Visually, the wall looked fine and there was no discoloration of the painted drywall (sheetrock). Upon closer examination, I could feel that the drywall was not dry. A foolish option would have been to take a hair dryer and a space heater and try to dry it out and have no concern about the possible underlying damage or mold growth. Obviously, overtime the rot would grow uncontrollably and who knows how much damage would eventually occur.

Clearly, no one would be foolish enough to use a hairdryer and space heater to deal with water damage in a wall...but that is representative of how people deal with chronic systemic body inflammation. I think this is the case because people do not properly conceptualize chronic inflammation as a state of systemic body rot.

Chronic inflammation means your body is rotting and it needs fixing
As stated in the beginning of this chapter, the problem is that "inflammation" has become a trivialized word and concept. Part of the trivialization process is related to the historical fact that people have been taking anti-inflammatory drugs for years.

The anti-inflammatory drugs I am referring to are aspirin and other non-steroidal anti-inflammatory drugs (NSAIDs), such as ibuprofen (Advil and Motrin) and naproxen (Aleve), which are available without a prescription. Examples of prescription NSAIDs include Celebrex, Feldene, Indocin, Naprosyn, Dolobid and many others.

By taking an "anti-inflammatory" drug, the human mind will believe that the drug will reduce inflammation and restore body function to normal. This belief is true for mild acute states of inflammation, such as minor joint and muscle aches and headaches. In contrast, this belief is completely false when it comes to chronic inflammation, which means a long-term state of body rot. Taking drugs or medications to reduce diet-induced chronic inflammation is actually no different an approach than using a hair dryer and space heater to fix a rotting, water-damaged wall.

If someone thinks, "my body has chronic inflammation," the natural follow-up thought is, "what can I take to reduce the inflammation?" The above-mentioned drugs would likely come to mind and there are a host of botanical products that are touted as natural anti-inflammatories, such as ginger, turmeric, and now CBD oil. People commonly tell me that they take these natural products to reduce their inflammation. Meanwhile, these same people are obviously rotting to me, as they are obese or overweight, and living with chronic life-limiting conditions like chronic pain, heart disease, diabetes, depression, cancer, and the list goes on. These people have chronic inflammatory conditions and do not understand what this type of inflammation really signifies.

What would most people think if I was to tell them that their bodies are actually and literally ROTTING? They would probably be confused…and might even think, "well I thought I only had inflammation, pain, and depression." No, the proper conceptualization should be that I am living in a mass of rotting flesh…OMG, what should I do about it?

The fact is that the presence of obesity, chronic pain, depression, heart disease, diabetes, cancer, etc., means that the body is biologically "rotting," and no drug or supplement can stop the rot.

> You should never again view chronic inflammation as anything other than chronic systemic body rot.

If, after reading the above information you were to properly think, "my body is biologically rotting and no drug or supplement can meaningfully help me," my question is this…what are you going to do?

My suggestion is to get mentally engaged with the information in this book. You need to properly understand the nature of chronic inflammation and view it properly as a state of ongoing "body rot," which can only be stopped and reversed by making appropriate lifestyle choices, the most notable being related to diet.

You first need a mental image of body rot. I will show you depictive images later in this book, but for now, you need to have a rotting concept in your mind. Fortunately, we have all been aware that things rot since we were kids. Everyone has witnessed food rotting. If you ever took a walk in the woods, you likely came upon a rotten tree log. We have all seen rusty old cars…they are rotting.

To "rot" simply means to decay. The most obvious example of the use of this term in healthcare is tooth decay…which really means tooth rot. How do you know if you have tooth rot? A dentist or hygienist will tell you as they examine your teeth during a routine visit, or you may feel pain when chewing. The cause of tooth decay is a pro-inflammatory diet and a lack of proper dental hygiene; both of which are easy to change.

It is unfortunate that this aspect of dental terminology has not been applied to other body conditions. Consider the fact that people with osteoarthritis are never told what the condition actually is, which is a state of "joint rot." The same rotting situation applies to degenerating and painful muscles, tendons, spinal discs, bones, and visceral (internal) organs. For example, osteoporosis is a state of chronic bone rot, which will be discussed in Chapter 18. The following are self-talk lifestyle messages to help prevent or reverse body rot.

- I need to eat well, so my body doesn't inflame and rot.
- I need to exercise regularly, so my body doesn't inflame and rot.
- I need to sleep well, so my body doesn't inflame and rot.
- I need to manage stress properly, so my body doesn't inflame and rot.
- I need to understand the nature of chronic inflammation so I do not trivialize the severity of the rotting process.

If people eat a pro-inflammatory diet, don't exercise, sleep poorly, and manage stress poorly, the most visible outcome will be weight gain. About 70% of the adult population in America is overweight or obese. In fact, almost 40% of adults are obese. As you will see in Chapter 10, obesity is a clear example of body rot chemistry that promotes rot throughout the entire body, which can be referred to as systemic body rot.

In short, any pro-inflammatory lifestyle choice that you make will add to the tidal wave of rot that is likely brewing in your body to some degree. For example, cigarette smoking and excess alcohol will also cause your body to rot.

The best way to get a handle on your personal body rot situation is to get easily measured inflammation markers into the normal range, which will be discussed in Chapter 3. Tracking these markers will allow you to maintain an even emotional state when it comes to your lifestyle choices. In other words, cheating is permitted so long as you keep your inflammation markers in the normal range.

Why you should embrace the body rot concept
I am writing these final few words in this introduction to emphasize that you should embrace the body rot concept of chronic inflammation. If you do that, you will be more likely to engage in healthy anti-inflammatory lifestyle choices because no one actually wants to suffer through their middle age and senior years in a state of chronic body rot that prevents one from enjoying life.

Chapter 1
The DeFlame Diet basics
Avoiding body rot chemistry

Body rot chemistry, called chronic inflammation, is known to be the cause of all chronic diseases, ranging from heart disease to cancer to depression to diabetes to osteoporosis and many more conditions. Chronic inflammation is also the cause of the musculoskeletal conditions that compromise most people to some degree, those being osteoarthritis, chronic joint pain, chronic muscle pain, spinal disc pain, and chronic tendon pain. You will discover in this book how these conditions represent a state of localized body rot (localized chronic inflammation), which is fed by a generalized state of systemic body rot chemistry (systemic chronic inflammation).

Figure 1 is a basic illustration of the key pro-inflammatory lifestyle factors that promote chronic inflammation and body rot. This simplified view should be quite understandable.

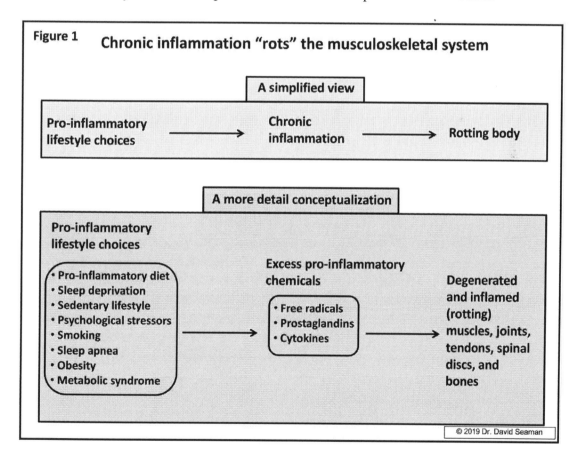

The more detailed conceptualization likely has some language that may be new to you. Perhaps the only pro-inflammatory lifestyle issue that you may not recognize is the metabolic syndrome, which is a pre-diabetic insulin resistant state. I will address this condition more in Chapters 3 and 12.

It is quite likely that you do not recognize all of the pro-inflammatory chemicals, which are important to understand and will be explained in this book so you do understand them. Free radicals are essentially pro-inflammatory oxidizing agents. Consider how old cars are commonly rusted and old looking. The rusting process is an oxidation process. In the human body, too many free radicals lead to body oxidation, inflammation, physical degeneration, and aging.

Prostaglandins are derived from dietary fats. The pro-inflammatory prostaglandins are derived from dietary omega-6 fatty acids. Consider the fact that many people take anti-inflammatory drugs like Advil (ibuprofen) on a daily basis to control their pain. The reason these medications help some people is because they inhibit the production of prostaglandins made from dietary omega-6 fatty acids. As was discussed in the introduction, these drugs do not address a chronic inflammatory state of body rot. When used on a daily basis, they serve to slightly reduce pain but do not address the excess dietary omega-6 fatty acids, which leads to a progression of body rot.

Cytokines are proteins that participate in the inflammatory process. Over 30 cytokines have been identified, most of which are pro-inflammatory. Save for a few, most cytokines are named based on their number. For example, the term interleukin refers to cytokines, which are numbered as interleukin-1 (IL-1), interleukin-2 (IL-2), and so on.

In this book, free radicals, prostaglandins, and cytokines will be described in Chapter 8 in a fashion that you will understand so that you can conceptualize how The DeFlame Diet can keep the production of these chemicals in the normal range to prevent our bodies from rotting. It is important to understand that we need these chemicals to be produced in proper amounts to support normal body functions. The same holds true for most body chemicals, which is why there are normal ranges for the various chemicals measured in a blood test. In the case of free radicals, prostaglandins, and cytokines, when they are produced in excess, the outcome is degeneration and inflammation of muscles, joints, tendons, discs and bones, i.e the rotting of musculoskeletal tissues.

Table 1 below was first published in *The DeFlame Diet* book, which is the most comprehensive book to date that outlines how diet promotes inflammation. The table below outlines pro-inflammatory calories versus DeFlame Diet options. Notice that you can make The DeFlame Diet ketogenic if you have an interest. The asterisks indicate the difference between a DeFlame Diet and a DeFlame Ketogenic Diet.

Table 1. Pro-inflammatory vs. DeFlame Diet vs. DeFlame Ketogenic Diet

Pro-inflammatory calories	DeFlame Diet	DeFlame Ketogenic Diet
Refined sugar	Grass-fed meat and wild game	Grass-fed meat and wild game
Refined grains	Meats	Meats
Grain flour products	Wild caught fish	Wild caught fish
Trans fats	Shellfish	Shellfish

Omega-6 seed oils (corn, safflower, sunflower, peanut, etc.)	Chicken	Chicken
	Omega-3 eggs	Omega-3 eggs
	Cheese	Cheese
	Vegetables	Vegetables
	Salads (leafy vegetables)	Salads (leafy vegetables)
	Fruit	* No fruit
	Roots/tubers (potato, yams, sweet potato)	* No roots/tubers
	Nuts (raw or dry roasted)	Nuts (raw or dry roasted)
	Omega-3 seeds: hemp, chia, flax seeds	Omega-3 seeds: hemp, chia, flax seeds
	Dark chocolate	* Sugar free dark chocolate
	Spices of all kinds	Spices of all kinds
	Olive oil, coconut oil, butter, cream, avocado, bacon	Olive oil, coconut oil, butter, cream, avocado, bacon
	Red wine and dark beer	Red wine
	Coffee and tea (green tea is best option)	Coffee and tea (green tea is best option)
		* No legumes and whole grains

Because of the abundance of books, blogs, websites, advertisements, etc., about nutrition, people tend to unnecessarily confuse and complicate how they view a healthy diet. Please notice in Table 1 the list of pro-inflammatory calories, which have no nutritional value; they only serve as a source of calories. Almost 60% of the average American's diet comes from these pro-inflammatory calories, which are implicated in the expression of all chronic diseases because eating these foods in excess will lead to an excessive production of free radicals, prostaglandins, and cytokines.

The guiding principle behind The DeFlame Diet is to normalize all the markers of inflammation, which are outlined in detail in Chapter 9 of *The DeFlame Diet* book. This means that one should not choose their foods based on an ideology, but rather based on your own biochemical needs and food preferences.

The first biochemical need that applies to EVERYONE is a proper caloric balance. Overeating is the key problem to avoid. No matter if one eats a vegan, omnivore, carnivore, Paleo, or ketogenic diet, calories can be over-consumed, which means that all of these diets can be pro-inflammatory.

Conversely, if the caloric balance is proper, all of these diets can be anti-inflammatory. The DeFlame Diet is NEVER pro-inflammatory, because the primary tenet is to achieve proper caloric balance. This is an especially important concept to understand, as overeating calories leads to chronic inflammation.

The challenge people have with giving up pro-inflammatory calories is that they taste really good and we crave them, which is why I use the term "dietary crack" to describe so-called "foods" made from sugar, flour, salt, and omega-6 oils (corn, safflower, sunflower, cottonseed, peanut, soybean oils). Breads, cakes, desserts, pretzels, donuts, French fries (and other deep-fried foods), oil roasted nuts, cereals, etc., are the most notable caloric culprits to be avoided. The easiest way to DeFlame your diet is to replace these calories with vegetation, which can rapidly lead to a normalization of all inflammatory markers.

The DeFlame Diet book is very inexpensive, at $9.99 for the Kindle book and $24.95 for paperback version.

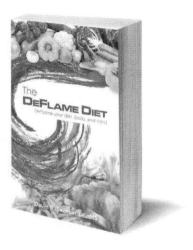

With the above information in mind, it should be understood that it is the cumulative effect of an excess consumption of the pro-inflammatory dietary factors that is the key issue. Eating a cookie every day at 100-200 calories would be irrelevant for the average person if all other pro-inflammatory factors in the diet were eliminated.

There is also a slippery slope to avoid at all costs that needs to be understood. People can maintain proper body weight on a diet of just French fries and donuts. In fact, you can be 100 pounds overweight and go on a 1000 calorie per day diet of just French fries and donuts and achieve a normal body weight. In this extreme case, you would achieve or maintain a normal body weight; however, you would be inflamed by an excess of omega-6 fatty acids from the oils used to make the French fries and donuts, as well as a lack of omega-3 fatty acids, magnesium, potassium, iodine, polyphenols, carotenoids, and other vitamins and minerals. The goal, as stated above, is to replace pro-inflammatory refined sugar, flour, and oil calories with vegetation.

The easiest way to begin the DeFlaming process

The easiest way to start DeFlaming is to reduce the number of hours spent each day eating, which is called time-restricted feeding (TRF). I think it is wise for everyone to fast at least 13 hrs per night and try to extend it up to 18 hours based on one's individual comfort level, and this is because TRF is exceptionally anti-inflammatory (1-4). Even if one eats the same pro-inflammatory calories, it is much better to do it in an 6-11 our eating window or less. Consider this real-life example.

I met a guy who told me that at the age 45 he was diagnosed with type 2 diabetes. At the time of the diagnosis his weight was 250 pounds, while his proper weight was 200 pounds. Because he did not want to take medications for the rest of his life, this man decided to eat just 600 calories per day within a 6-hr time period until he got his weight back to 200 lbs. For 3 months he ate a double cheeseburger from MacDonald's, which was about 450 calories. The remaining 150 calories were from vegetables and fruit. At the end of the 3 months, he weighed 200 pounds again and no longer had diabetes.

I am not suggesting that anyone should do the double cheeseburger plan. The point of this example is to illustrate that there are many ways to DeFlame. My suggestion is to drastically avoid refined sugar, flour, and oils whether one chooses to be a vegan, omnivore, or carnivore and then let the normalization of inflammatory markers be the ultimate eating guide. In most cases, it is not a requirement for the diet to be ketogenic, so go keto only if it suits your individual preferences. Whichever foods you choose to eat, begin with a 13-hr fast and then extend it based on your comfort level, which can vary day to day.

References

1. Marinack CR, Nelson SH, Breen CI, et al. Prolonged nightly fasting and breast cancer prognosis. JAMA Oncol. 2016;2:1049-55.
2. Moro T, Tinsley G, Bianco A, et al. Effects of eight weeks of time-restricted feeding (16/8) on basal metabolism, maximal strength, body composition, inflammation, and cardiovascular risk factors in resistance-trained males. J Translational Med. 2016;14:290.
3. Jamshed H, Beyl RA, Della Manna DL, et al. Early time-restricted feeding improves 24-hour glucose levels and affects markers of the circadian clock, aging, and autophagy in humans. Nutrients. 2019;11:1234.
4. de Cabo R, Mattson MP. Effects of intermittent fasting on health, aging, and disease. New Eng J Med. 2019;381:2541-51.

Chapter 2
The diet-related chemicals that rot the body

In Chapter 1, you were introduced to the basics of the pro-inflammatory chemistry that rots the body. Free radicals, prostaglandins, and cytokines are the big players in the rotting process; however, there are more rot-promoting chemicals that you need to be aware of as you read through this book. This chapter will essentially function as a glossary of terms for the various chemicals that rot our visceral (internal) organs and musculoskeletal tissues.

Each of the headings in this chapter is a question, which is followed by the answer that you should understand by the time you finish this book. In other words, in this chapter, the basics will be discussed and in later chapters more details will be added.

What are free radicals and how do they rot my body?

Free radicals are essentially pro-inflammatory oxidizing agents. Consider how old cars are commonly rusted and old looking. The rusting process is an oxidation process. In the human body, too many free radicals lead to body oxidation, inflammation, physical degeneration, and aging. Whether the oxidation is taking place in a rusty old car or in a flaming human body, it should be viewed as a rotting process. Our cells produce an excess of free radicals, which rot the body, when they are exposed to a pro-inflammatory diet rich in refined sugar, flour, and oils.

What are prostaglandins and how do they rot my body?

Prostaglandins are hormone-like substances that are derived from dietary fats. The pro-inflammatory prostaglandins are derived from dietary omega-6 fatty acids. Consider the fact that many people take anti-inflammatory drugs like Advil (ibuprofen) on a daily basis to control their pain. It turns out that these medications inhibit the production of prostaglandins made from dietary omega-6 fatty acids. An excess of prostaglandin production is associated with inflammation and body tissue degeneration, which means the body is rotting.

What are omega-6 fatty acids and how do they rot my body?

The abbreviation for omega-6 is n-6, so you will often see n-6 fatty acids and you should know that this means omega-6 fatty acids. The first thing to know is that fats are made up of fatty acids. In other words, the fat in meat, fish, nuts, avocados, olive oil and all other foods is made up of saturated fatty acids, monounsaturated fatty acids, and polyunsaturated fatty acids.

The polyunsaturated fatty acids can either be omega-6 or omega-3 (also referred to as n-3). The difference being the location of the first double bond nearest to the omega carbon, which I understand makes no sense to you unless you understand fatty acid structures. If you wish to learn more about this, you can search the internet for fatty acid structures or you can get *The DeFlame Diet* book, which goes over the details.

For our purposes here and now, you need to know that we are supposed to have a ratio of n-6:n-3 of less than 4 to 1. We can achieve this by eating The DeFlame Diet and taking omega-3 fatty acid supplements. This does require us to eliminate completely, or keep to a bare minimum, the consumption of processed and deep fried foods that contain refined oils rich in omega-6 fatty acids. The refined oils to eliminate from your diet are from corn, safflower, sunflower, cottonseed, grape seed, peanut, and soybeans.

Eating an excess of n-6 fatty acids will cause body cells to produce excessive amount of pro-inflammatory prostaglandins. The same n-6 fatty acid excess also leads to an excess production of pro-inflammatory cytokines. This means that n-6 fatty acids rot the body via an excessive production of pro-inflammatory prostaglandins and cytokines.

What are cytokines and how do they rot my body?
Cytokines are proteins that participate in the inflammatory process and when chronically produced in excess, they rot the body. Over 30 cytokines have been identified, most of which are pro-inflammatory. Save for a few, most cytokines are named based on their number. For example, the term interleukin refers to cytokines, which are numbered as interleukin-1, interleukin-2, and so on. Overeating refined sugar, flour, and oils, causes body cells to produce an excess of pro-inflammatory cytokines, which rot the body.

What is hyperglycemia and how does it rot my body?
Hyperglycemia means too much glucose in the body, which can be easily determined with a blood test or at home with a glucometer. Hyperglycemia is caused by an overconsumption of refined sugar and flour, which are also referred to as refined carbohydrates. A shocking 40% of the dietary calories consumed by Americans come from refined sugar and flour. The metabolic syndrome and type 2 diabetes are conditions in which the body perpetually exists in a hyperglycemic state. The outcome is that cells exposed to hyperglycemia produce an excess of free radicals, prostaglandins, and cytokines, which cause the body to rot.

What is insulin and how does it rot my body?
Insulin is released by cells in the pancreas when blood glucose levels rise after a meal. It is important to understand that, historically speaking, humans ate no refined carbohydrates for the vast majority of our time on earth; we only ate whole foods, so there was never a dramatic rise in blood glucose after a meal until refined carbohydrates were created by man. This means that insulin levels never rose above normal until refined carbohydrates were produced by man and then overconsumed by the population.

Over time, as refined carbohydrates are consumed in excess and body fat mass accumulates, the population began to develop type 2 diabetes, which is a state of both high blood glucose (hyperglycemia) and high blood insulin (hyperinsulinemia).

Excess insulin is the key issue that leads to the overproduction of cholesterol and body fat, which causes the body to rot. This will be discussed in Chapter 12 (Metabolic syndrome) and Chapter 13 (Atherosclerosis).

What is oxidized LDL cholesterol (ox-LDL) and how does it rot my body?

While essentially everyone has heard of LDL cholesterol, most people have never heard of oxidized LDL (oxLDL) cholesterol. It will be discussed in more detail in Chapter 13, but for now, here is a bit of introductory information.

LDL cholesterol has been portrayed to be "bad" cholesterol, which is only the case if it is free radicalized to become oxLDL by a pro-inflammatory diet. In other words, normal LDL cholesterol does not cause heart disease or any other condition. In contrast, oxLDL is pro-inflammatory and a key driver of atherosclerotic vascular disease, as well as musculoskeletal conditions, because it stimulates the immune system. The outcome is chronic inflammation and body rot.

What is ox-HDL and how does it rot my body?

In contrast with LDL cholesterol, HDL cholesterol is referred to as our good cholesterol. This too is a misnomer. HDL cholesterol is good only if it has not become free radicalized to become oxidized HDL (oxHDL) cholesterol. Just like LDL, a pro-inflammatory diet causes HDL cholesterol to become oxidized. Once oxidized, HDL cholesterol is no longer able to function in an anti-inflammatory fashion to prevent body rot.

What are triglycerides, diglycerides, palmitic acid, and ceramide, and how do they rot my body?

Triglycerides, diglycerides, palmitic acid, and ceramide are fats. If you ever looked at your blood test results, you saw triglycerides, which is the body's way to store fats. Lean, athletic people have normal levels of triglycerides, which means that triglycerides are not inherently pro-inflammatory. In contrast, a high triglyceride level is a marker of chronic inflammation and is associated with obesity, the metabolic syndrome, and type 2 diabetes.

As stated above, lean, healthy bodies have triglycerides; however, a healthy body does not accumulate pro-inflammatory diglycerides, palmitic acid, and ceramide. The term "lipotoxicity" is used to characterize a body that is storing these pro-inflammatory fats.

Diglycerides represent an abnormal form of fat storage that occurs in people with obesity, the metabolic syndrome, and type 2 diabetes. Palmitic acid is a saturated fatty acid that is produced in excess in the liver and fat cells when refined sugar and flour are consumed in excess, which is the case for most Americans. Excess palmitic acid itself is pro-inflammatory and some of the excess is converted into a pro-inflammatory fat called ceramide. This pattern of lipotoxicity is especially obvious in skeletal muscle and will be discussed in more detail in Chapter 14.

What are pro-inflammatory immune cells and how do they rot my body?
The human body contains different types of immune cells. Some are pro-inflammatory and the others are anti-inflammatory, and there needs to be a balance between the two. This balance is lost as people become obese, and favors an excess of pro-inflammatory immune cells, which rot the body by preventing proper healing and promoting chronic inflammation. This pro-inflammatory shift in immune function will be illustrated in several chapters in this book.

What is endotoxin and how does it rot my body?
Endotoxin, also known as lipopolysaccharide, is found in the outer cell wall of gram-negative bacteria. About half of the bacteria in the human gut are gram-negative and the other half are gram-positive. When we overeat refined sugar, flour, and oils, an excess of endotoxin is released by gram-negative bacteria, which is then absorbed through the gut wall and gets into body circulation. Subsequently, body cells that are exposed to an excess of endotoxin will release cytokines and other inflammatory mediators, which cause the body to rot.

What are AGEs and how do they rot my body?
AGEs is the acronym for advanced glycation end products. They accumulate in the body as a consequence of living in a state of chronic hyperglycemia. Glycation refers to the binding of glucose to body proteins and lipids (fats), which are then termed advanced glycation end products (AGEs).

Hemoglobin is a protein and excess glucose in circulation binds to hemoglobin. Hemoglobin A1c is the most well-known of the AGEs and reflects glucose levels for the previous 120 days. Excess glucose also binds to lipids, such as LDL cholesterol. Additional AGEs are created in the body due to hyperglycemia, such as pentosidine, carboxymethyllysine and carboxyethyllysine. An excess of AGEs is known to promote chronic inflammation and body rot.

AGEs also come preformed in foods and so they are called dietary AGEs. There are relatively few dietary AGEs in vegetables, fruits, whole grains, legumes, and milk. In contrast, animal products, which consist of protein and fat, are high in dietary AGEs.

Cooking animal products with dry heat methods (broiling, roasting, grilling, and frying) can increase content of dietary AGEs by 10 to 100 times (1,2). This is part of the reason why radical vegan groups incorrectly claim that eating any animal products at all is pro-inflammatory and disease-promoting. If this were true, then the Maasai tribe in Kenya would have been the sickest population of people on earth. The traditional diet of the Maasai consisted of meat, blood, and milk; HOWEVER, this population of people was remarkably healthy and free of the chronic diseases that have crippled industrialized nations like the United States. So, if eating meat, blood, and milk did not cause disease in the Maasai, there is no way that eating a traditional omnivore diet of animal products and vegetation could possibly cause disease. Unfortunately, radical vegan groups are unable to embrace this fact.

As stated in Chapter 1, you can DeFlame your body by eating a vegan, omnivore, or carnivore diet. The key is for the diet to be calorically appropriate and virtually free of pro-inflammatory refined sugar, flour, and oil calories, which were never consumed by native people anywhere on earth until the modern age. When we overeat these pro-inflammatory calories, the outcome is obesity and hyperglycemia. As stated above, hyperglycemia causes AGE production in the body, which can be readily tracked by testing for hemoglobin A1c.

In the case of dietary AGEs, the human body has a natural system for their elimination. In short, dietary AGEs bind to the AGE receptor-1 on liver and immune cells, which leads to the elimination of dietary AGEs so they do not cause inflammation (3,4). Thus, the AGE receptor-1 can be viewed as the anti-inflammatory receptor AGEs. There is also a pro-inflammatory "Receptor for AGEs," and it is referred to as RAGE. Inflammation is induced when AGEs bind to RAGE.

When people become hyperglycemic and diabetic, a condition called fatty liver develops, which is associated with a reduction in anti-inflammatory AGE receptor-1 levels and an increase in RAGE levels (3,4). Additionally, a hormone called leptin, which is produced in excess by obese fat cells, also reduces anti-inflammatory AGE receptor-1 levels and an increase in RAGE levels (4). When this happens, the human body is not able to properly eliminate dietary AGEs, so they accumulate and cause chronic inflammation.

In short, the average American is overweight or obese, which means that people consume an excess of calories and we know these calories come from refined sugar, flour, and oils. Indeed, the average American gets 40% of their calories from refined sugar and flour, and they consume animal products with an excess of AGEs. This means that these people produce an excess of AGEs in their own bodies, the most notable being hemoglobin A1c, and simultaneously reduce their ability to clear AGEs from the body. They also overeat dietary AGEs, which adds to the burden AGE-induced inflammation.

The only way to normalize A1c levels other body-produced AGEs is to normalize fasting and postprandial glucose by DeFlaming the diet. This will allow anti-inflammatory AGE receptor-1 and pro-inflammatory RAGE levels to return to normal. The next step is to reduce the consumption of dietary AGEs, which is easier than you may think. First, avoid all deep-fried and processed foods. Second, modify how meat is cooked. Believe it or not, you can still broil, roast, grill, and fry animal products. However, they should be first marinated in lemon juice, vinegar, or any other acidic marinade, which significantly reduces the AGEs produced during dry heat cooking. Lower cooking temperatures also reduces AGE production. Several herbs are potent inhibitors of AGE production, such as sage, marjoram, tarragon, rosemary, cloves, ground Jamaican allspice, and cinnamon (2). Alternative methods of cooking can reduce AGE production by 50%, those being boiling and stewing (2).

Here is how I have cooked animal products for many years. I only eat grass-fed chopped meat at home, which I slowly cook in a pan on the stove, which means it is not a dry heat method that increases AGEs. I also add a lot of spices to the meat. I buy only hormone-free bacon and also slowly cook it, and then eat it with a pound or more of vegetation with added spices. I cook fish and chicken in a pan on the stove top and cook it in water with a variety of spices. Regarding fish, I only eat wild caught varieties and mostly stick with salmon. For chicken, I buy only free range and hormone-free.

As you have read, I cook animal products in a fashion that will not augment AGE production. I almost never cook with oils or butter, and if I do, it is at a relatively low temperature that does not cause the oil or butter to burn. Finally, since my blood glucose levels are normal, I have not disrupted the anti-AGE activity of the AGE receptor-1, so the odds that dietary AGEs are causing a problem for omnivores like me are minimal.

Final thoughts

A common question emerges after people read the above information. They want to know what they can take to block the activity of the various inflammatory chemicals. The answer is:

> There is nothing you can take; you have to eat an anti-inflammatory diet and return your body physiology back to an anti-inflammatory state.

In the following chapter, the basics of how to track inflammation (body rot) will be described. If the markers of inflammation are normal, then the various inflammatory chemicals discussed in this chapter will normalize.

In subsequent chapters, you will see these pro-inflammatory chemicals appear again and again as the key culprits in the body rot process that trashes the vascular system and musculoskeletal tissues. I have created images so you can visualize how these chemicals rot arteries, muscles, joints, tendons, spinal discs, and bones.

References

1. Uribarri J, Woodruff S, Goodman S, et al. Advanced glycation end products in foods and a practical guide to their reduction in the diet. J Am Diet Assoc. 2010;110:911-16.
2. Abate G, Debarba A, Marziano M, et al. Advanced glycation end products (AGEs) in food: focusing on Mediterranean pasta. J Nutr Food Sci. 2015;5:6.
3. Vlassara H, Cai W, Goodman S, et al. Protection against loss of innate defenses in adulthood by low advanced glycation end products (AGE) intake: role of anti-inflammatory AGE receptor-1. J Clin Endocrinol Metab. 2009;94:4483-91.
4. Tang Y, Chen A. Curcumin eliminates the effect of advanced glycation end-products (AGEs) on the divergent regulation of gene expression of receptors of AGEs by interrupting leptin signaling. Lab Invest. 2014;94:503-16.

Chapter 3
Tracking inflammation
How you know if your body is rotting

Tracking inflammatory markers is very easy when you are older and obviously inflamed. It is not so straightforward when you are young and basically fit. The problem for many young people is that they cannot visualize, or do not want to visualize, themselves as their future older and rotting self, who will likely be inflamed and in pain if they do not take care of their younger selves. The easiest way for young athletes and active people to embrace The DeFlame Diet is to accept the fact that overeating sugar, flour, and refined omega-6 oils will gradually inflame and rot the musculoskeletal tissues (muscles, joints, tendons, and bones) that allow us to engage in physical activities. I will describe this in more detail in Chapters 14-18.

For those people who have aged beyond youthfulness, inflammation tracking is quite simple to do. For example, it turns out that an elevated waist/hip ratio correlates closely with inflammation and degeneration of our musculoskeletal tissues. This is because abdominal fat accumulation correlates with the development of chronic inflammation, which is outlined in Chapter 10. Measuring waist/hip ratio is very simple to do and correlates with common markers of inflammation, such as blood pressure and blood markers, including glucose, triglycerides, HDL cholesterol, and C-reactive protein.

Waist circumference is measured at the umbilicus (belly button), which typically reflects the greatest area of abdominal girth, and thus, the presence or absence of abdominal obesity. For some people, the greatest abdominal girth is an inch above or an inch below the umbilicus. You want to measure where you have the most abdominal girth. You then divide the waist circumference by hip circumference.

The hip measurement should be done in a fashion to capture the most mass of the buttocks, which you typically find at the level of the greater trochanter (see image on next page). You find the greater trochanter at the top of the thigh bone. The greater trochanter is large and sticks out, so it is easy to feel. Put your hands on your buttocks, then slide them to the side and you will fill the greater trochanter of the thigh bone. Measure your hip circumference where you feel the greater trochanter.

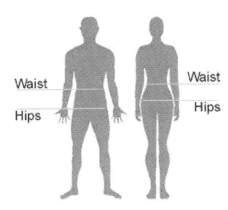

A normal waist/hip ratio for women is .8, which indicates that the waist measure should be less than the hip measurement. Anything higher than .8 reflects a gradual increase in ongoing inflammation and body rot.

A normal waist/hip ratio for men is .95, which again, indicates that the waist measure should be less than the hip measurement. Anything higher than .95 reflects a gradual increase in ongoing inflammation and body rot.

If you want to directly measure inflammation, you can ask your doctor to do a blood test to measure C-reactive protein (CRP). As the name suggests, CRP is an inflammatory protein that rises and falls based on inflammatory stimuli. For example, in a young, lean and healthy adult, CRP will rise during a sickness, such as the common cold, and then fall back to normal after the cold goes away. If CRP levels are high when one is not "sick," this likely indicates a chronic inflammatory state of body rot.

CRP is produced by the liver in response to increasing levels of cytokines, particularly interleukin-6, (IL-6). For most readers of this book, cytokines and IL-6 will have no meaning for you, so this topic should be viewed as a learning moment. As stated in Chapter 1, cytokines are proteins that participate in the inflammatory process. Over 30 cytokines have been identified, most of which are pro-inflammatory. Interleukins are a family of cytokines, of which IL-6 is a member. When IL-6 levels rise above normal, it stimulates the liver to overproduce CRP.

A normal CRP level is below 1.0 mg/L, which should be the goal for all of us and reflects a rot-free state in the body. An individual is considered to be moderately rotting (inflamed) if their CRP level is between 1-3 mg/L. The average adult American has a CRP level of 1.5 mg/L, which means the average adult in America spends 24 hours per day in a state of moderate rot. If CRP levels rise above 3 mg/L, the individual is considered to be highly inflamed. It turns out that about 25% of adult Americans have CRP levels above 3 mg/L (1), which means that a substantial part of the US population is aggressively rotting.

Table 1 contains the markers used to identify the metabolic syndrome, which is a pro-inflammatory state of body rot that promotes chronic diseases like heart disease, cancer, and diabetes. This same syndrome also promotes muscle, joint, tendon, bone, and spinal disc degeneration, which will be discussed more in Chapters 14-18.

Table 1 - Metabolic syndrome markers

Metabolic syndrome	Abnormal value	Date	Date	Date	Date
1. Fasting blood glucose	≥ 100 mg/dL				
2. Fasting triglycerides	≥ 150 mg/dL				
3. Fasting HDL cholesterol	< 50 for women; < 40 men				
4. Blood pressure	≥ 130/85				
5. Waist circumference	> 35" women; > 40" men				

In order to be diagnosed with the metabolic syndrome, you need at least 3 of the 5 markers to have an abnormal value. Approximately 25% of all adults in the United States have the metabolic syndrome. This number rises to about 45% of adults over the age of 60 (2,3), which demonstrates how pervasive the state of body rot is in the American population.

As I am writing this book, I have completed year 59 and am just beginning my 60th year. If I want the best chance to have healthy muscles, joints, tendons and bones, my waist/hip ratio should be below .95, CRP should be below 1 mg/L, and I should have no abnormal values for markers of the metabolic syndrome.

For a much larger list of inflammation markers that you can track, my suggestion is to get a copy of *The DeFlame Diet* book, which addresses a wide array of diet-inflammation issues to a much greater degree than in this book. The purpose of this book is to focus mostly on how diet-induced chronic inflammation causes our musculoskeletal tissues to rot and compromise our physical function.

References
1. Ridker PM. Cardiology patient page. C-reactive protein: a simple test to help predict risk of heart attack and stroke. Circulation 2003, 108:81–85.
2. Ford ES, Giles WH, Dietz WH. Prevalence of the metabolic syndrome among US adults. Findings from the Third National Health and Nutrition Examination Survey. J Am Med Assoc. 200; 287:356-59.
3. Ford ES. Prevalence of the metabolic syndrome defined by the International Diabetes Federation among adults in the U.S. Diabetes Care. 2005;28(11):2745-49.

Chapter 4
Accepting the fact that you are rotting

If you are reading this book, it is likely due to the fact that you are rotting. Or, you are concerned about your health and do not want to rot. Either way, we all must accept the fact that our bodies will rot and suffer the consequences if we make poor lifestyle choices.

When people are young and fit, they can eat almost anything and feel fine, so most young people do not give good nutrition a second thought. It was a little different for me. In my senior year of high school, I was already moving in the direction of health and fitness, and nutrition was an interest of mine. I hardly ever drank soda and mostly controlled my dessert intake; and more importantly, I understood that these calories served no benefit to my health so I kind of felt a little guilty when I ate them; however, I never felt unwell. With this in mind, during my senior year of high school, a buddy and I decided we would bicycle from our town in New Jersey to Florida. We actually managed to pull this trip off; our parents let us do it and we arrived at our Florida destination in about 20 days. We could have made it faster, but it rained every day the first week, so the going was initially very, very slow, as we peddled along wearing our ponchos.

In order for me to able to afford the trip, I had to get some money together and also save up money to cover expenses for my freshman year of college. So, during the latter part of my senior year in high school, I bussed tables at a popular restaurant. This involved 8-10 hours during a night and we typically finished up close to midnight, or thereafter. My feet typically hurt after an evening because the shoes I wore were not the most comfortable. When time permitted, we would get a meal and we could drink water or soda from the fountain we had in the bus stations.

One Friday night of bussing was particularly long and busy. I recollect eating a burger with fries and drank soda on-and-off during the night…not at all the DeFlame approach to diet that I eventually began to understand many years later. I had to be up early the next morning for our county track and field championship; I was a high jumper. My father was going to go, but I told him that since I had not been doing that great during senior year and because of so little sleep, I would probably bomb.

When I got home, I had to tell my dad that I won the event with a personal best of 6'6". On a side note, I was never able to jump any higher in college, but my father came to one event and saw me clear 6'6". An injury in my sophomore year of college sidelined me and I never competed again. But the point of this story was how impressed I was even then that I could perform so well in the county championship on so little sleep and with an eating style that I would now characterize as not very anti-inflammatory.

To me, this is an example of how youth is wasted on the young. In short, when we are young, we have not lived long enough for our bodies to go through the rotting process. For this reason, when we are young, we are naturally very resilient and can handle acute bouts of sleep loss, too much drinking, and regularly eating "flamey" foods. Unfortunately, the subconscious mind takes note of this and propels us into living this way in our more sedentary working years after college until retirement age. Most people continue to eat the same amount and types of calories despite engaging in less physical activity. The outcome is that most people put on weight and progressively lose the youthful feeling they had in their high school and college years; the body begins to rot. If we continue on this pro-inflammatory path, it is common to develop physical aches and pains, gut troubles, depression, hypertension, etc., as early as in our 30s and 40s, which can continue for the rest of our lives, and eventually manifest as diabetes, a heart attack or stroke, and cancer.

If you are still young, fit, and resilient, the information in this book represents an accurate picture of your future decline of musculoskeletal and general health if you eat a pro-inflammatory diet as you age. If you are in your 30s or older, your musculoskeletal system may already be rotting due to consuming a pro-inflammatory diet. Most people who hit their 50s and 60s look back and wish they treated their bodies better when they were young. I cannot tell you how many people in their 50s and older tell me that they wish they ate better the past 30 years of their lives.

A problem for our minds when it comes to unhealthy behaviors when we are young is that we typically do not make a cause-effect correlation between poor health choices when we are young and a poor health outcome in the future. Our emotional brain literally thinks that if we eat tasty pro-inflammatory calories when we are young and we do not develop pain, depression, etc., this means that we can continue the same unhealthy eating for the rest of our lives...in fact, our emotional brain is quite wrong, so we need to learn to override our emotional desires for tasty pro-inflammatory foods when we are young.

It is important to understand that many people reach a point when they can no longer tolerate large doses of pro-inflammatory foods. I used to occasionally grab lunch with a colleague, who was probably about 50 years old at that time. He would always get wings and fries, both of which are obviously deep-fried in omega-6 oils. After lunch one day, he told me that every time he eats that type of meal, his hands stiffen up, hurt, and feel arthritic. We can learn two important points from this example. First, this guy reached a state of body rot that became overtly symptomatic by merely eating wings and fries. Second, he clearly realized the cause-effect scenario, but nonetheless continued to keep eating the same foods. This speaks to the power of tasty pro-inflammatory calories; we are literally mesmerized and controlled by them, even when they cause immediate and obvious symptoms of body rot.

Unless one has an acute inflammatory reaction to a meal, as described above, it is fine for most people to enjoy pro-inflammatory calories on an occasional basis, but we have to learn how to control what I call the "eating beast within," which gets mesmerized and controlled by these calories. In order to prevent the development of inflammatory food-related diseases as we age, we have to exert control over our eating environment, our primordial drives to overeat, and our emotions. This is actually the topic of my book entitled, *Weight Loss Secrets You Need To Know*. If you read it when you are lean and healthy, it will help you stay lean and healthy. If you are an overweight flamer, it will help you to become lean and healthy and prevent systemic body rot.

Unfortunately for some, the dietary "flame" can strike people when they are in their teens or younger. Consider the fact that asthma and eczema are very common in the young population and have all been linked to the overconsumption of refined sugar, flour, and oil calories, and we have known about this since at least as early as the year 2000 (1-8). This means that many of our young children are unnecessarily rotting.

Understanding your body - your inflammation status
No matter how flamed up you are, you need to accept it, stare your situation in the face, and work to DeFlame yourself and hopefully set yourself free from whatever degree of rot you are currently experiencing. If you are not obviously rotting, you should use the information in this book as a preventive measure so you never land in the state of chronic pain and depression, or worse, diabetes, heart disease, cancer, or Alzheimer's disease.

Of course, the flame will win and we will all die eventually. However, by understanding the enemy (chronic inflammation) we can engage in activities to minimize the rotting damage, which will allow us to live longer lives without pain, physical disability, and chronic disease.

In upcoming chapters, I will describe the rotting changes that occur in muscles, joints, tendons, spinal discs, and bones when we flame up. The first action step you should take to DeFlame and improve the quality of your musculoskeletal tissues is to identify your levels of the inflammation markers discussed in Chapter 3. You need to accept the fact that you are rotting or will rot if you are not careful...and do this from a positive perspective, meaning that you can reverse the rot if you DeFlame your diet. In the next chapter, the topic of inflammaging will be described, which is another dimension of body rot that should be understood.

References
1. Hijazi N et al. Diet and childhood asthma in a society in transition: a study in urban and rural Saudi Arabia. Thorax. 2000;55:775-79.
2. Smit HA et al. Chronic obstructive pulmonary disease, asthma and protective effects of food intake: from hypothesis to evidence. Respir Res 2001;2:261-64.
3. Mellis CM. Is asthma prevention possible with dietary manipulation? Med J Aust. 2002;177:S78-S80.
4. McKeever TM, Britton J. Diet and asthma. Am J Respir Crit Care Med. 2004; 170:725-29.
5. Chatzi L et al. Mediterranean Diet in pregnancy protective for wheeze and atopy in childhood. Thorax. 2008;63:507-13.
6. Chatzi L et al. Protective effect of fruits, vegetables and the Mediterranean diet on asthma and allergies among children in Crete.Thorax. 2007;62:677-83.
7. Chatzi L et al. Diet, wheeze, and atopy in school children in Menorca, Spain.Pediatr Allergy Immunol. 2007;18:480-85

8. Ellwood P, Asher MI, Garcia-Marcos L, et al. Do fast foods cause asthma, rhinoconjunctivitis, and eczema? Global findings from the International Study of Asthma and Allergies in Childhood (ISAAC) Phase Three. Thorax. 2013;68:351-60.

Chapter 5
Inflammaging and your muscles, joints, tendons, bones, and skin

Our goal should be to live in a rot-free state as we age. In scientific terms, this means we should inflammage properly.

Inflammaging refers to the normal inflammatory changes that occur with aging. Inflammaging is unavoidable because we are all aging. Despite this fact, we need not suffer the ravages of dramatic pro-inflammatory inflammaging if we make the right lifestyle choices. Scientist tell us that we can either anti-inflammage or pro-inflammage (1-9). My suggestion, obviously, is to anti-inflammage, which means normal inflammaging. Normal inflammaging means that an old body wears out *without* rotting. Pro-inflammaging means that the body lives in state of body rot that is associated with years of rotting misery.

If you are young and fit or relatively fit, it is difficult to conceptualize the inflammaging process. All you need to do is look around and you will see that most people are pro-inflammaging, which means that they literally look like they are rotting. Most adult Americans are overweight or obese and taking medications for blood sugar, blood pressure, cholesterol, and other conditions. These same people are physically deconditioned and unable to engage in activities that leaner versions of themselves could easily handle. The pro-inflammagers also move slowly without any vim and vigor. Their skin looks too old, wrinkled, and sagging for their age. In short, people often look 10 or more years older than they are. The way to avoid this is to understand that it will happen to you if you adopt a pro-inflammatory lifestyle, which means you must instead adopt a DeFlaming lifestyle.

I occasionally run into exceptionally fit women and men in their 50s and 60s. This is a rare breed of people, but they do exist. They age gracefully even though they are still inflammaging, which means they preserve proper musculoskeletal function far longer than the average pro-inflammager who is rotting away.

For most people who were once young and fit, the pro-inflammaging process often occurs at an unexpectedly rapid pace. Between the ages of 25 and 50, most people are focused on making a living and supporting a family, both of which can be stressful. Stress leads to sedentary living and overeating, and before one knows it, they are obese and may also have chronic pain, depression and/or anxiety. I have personally witnessed this transformation in many people who had no expectation of it ever happening to them.

If you are already in a pro-inflammaging state, you need to reverse it as soon as possible to protect your musculoskeletal tissues. The best way to properly inflammage is to follow The DeFlame Diet, exercise, get adequate sleep, avoid unnecessary financial and emotional stressors, learn to manage the stressors that you cannot avoid, don't smoke, don't drink alcohol in excess, and engage in relationships that are supportive and nurturing. All of this is easier said than done, but nonetheless, it is the path to healthy inflammaging, which will preserve the health of your musculoskeletal tissues so you can engage in your favorite physical activities.

References

1. Franceschi C, Bonafe M, Valensin S et al. Inflamm-aging. An evolutionary perspective on immunosenescence. Ann N Y Acad Sci. 2000; 908:244-54

2. De Martinis M, Franceschi C et al. Inflamm-ageing and lifelong antigenic load as major determinants of ageing rate and longevity. FEBS Lett. 2005 ;579(10):2035-9

3. Franceschi C. Inflammaging as a major characteristic of old people: can it be prevented or cured? Nutr Rev. 2007;65(12 Pt 2):S173-6

4. Franceschi C, Capri M, Monti D, et al. Inflammaging and anti-inflammaging: a systemic perspective on aging and longevity emerged from studies in humans. Mech Ageing Dev. 2007;128:92–105.

5. Hunt KJ, Walsh FB, Voegeli D, Roberts HC. Inflammation in aging Part 1: physiology and immunological mechanisms. Biol Res Nurs. 2010;11(3):245-52.

6. Hunt KJ, Walsh FB, Voegeli D, Roberts HC. Inflammation in aging Part 2: implications for the health of older people and recommendations for nursing practice. Biol Res Nurs. 2010;11(3):253-60/.

7. Xia S, Zhang X, Zheng S, et al. An update on inflamm-aging: mechanisms, prevention, and treatment. J Immunol Res. 2016;2016:8426874.

8. Franceschi C, Garagnani P, Parini P, Giuliani C, Santor A. Inflammaging: a new immune-metabolic viewpoint for age-related diseases. Nature Rev Endocrinol. 2018;14:576-90.

9. Franceshi C, Garagnani P, Vitale G, Capri M, Salvioli S. Inflammaging and 'garb-aging'. Trends Endocrinol Metab. 2017;28:199-212.

Chapter 6
Diet and pain expression

Pain expression refers to the emergence of pain. Most people who have aches and pains cannot remember a specific event that caused them to convert from a pain-free state to one that is painful. Chronic pain most commonly emerges or expresses itself over time in a cumulative fashion that does not allow for one to identify a specific event that definitively led to the manifestation of pain.

In the absence of an identifiable injury, chronic pain typically emerges as a consequence of living a pro-inflammatory lifestyle that is characterized by a lack of sleep, ongoing stress, sedentary living, and a pro-inflammatory diet. Obviously, the topic of this book is about how our diet can cause us to "flame up" and rot, and develop chronic pain. I described this process in detail in *The DeFlame Diet* book and in these articles found in the references of this chapter (1-4). Herein, I will describe an abbreviated and simplified version of acute and chronic dietary inflammation as outlined in Figures 1 & 2.

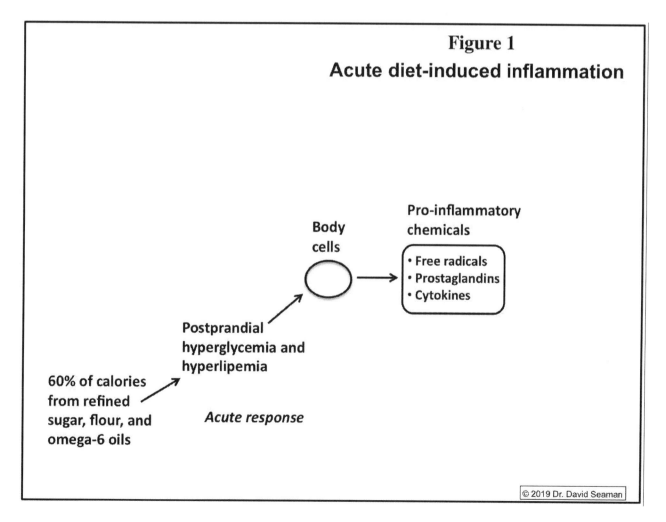

Figure 1
Acute diet-induced inflammation

Body cells

Pro-inflammatory chemicals
- Free radicals
- Prostaglandins
- Cytokines

Postprandial hyperglycemia and hyperlipemia

60% of calories from refined sugar, flour, and omega-6 oils

Acute response

© 2019 Dr. David Seaman

If you are living in a DeFlamed state, a random pro-inflammatory pig-out session will only cause a short-lived increase in pro-inflammatory chemicals, which is certainly not enough to cause body rot. The biggest pro-inflammatory dietary issue for most Americans is chronically overeating refined sugar, flour, and refined omega-6 oils, which leads to weight and obesity. These calories are typically derived from desserts, chips, bread, French fries, and similar so-called foods. In the case of sugar, it is found in processed foods and also added directly to various foods and drinks by people at home and at restaurants. It turns out that the average American consumes about 150 pounds of refined sugar per year.

Approximately 40% of all calories consumed by Americans come from refined sugar and flour products, and 20% comes from refined oils. Figure 1 outlines what happens after we eat a large dose of these calories.

No matter what age we are, whenever we pig-out on these calories, which is a daily event for most people, there is a postprandial (after eating) rise in blood levels of glucose (hyperglycemia) and fat (hyperlipemia). The same thing would happen if no oils or fats were consumed and we just ate "foods" made of refined sugar and/or flour. The outcome is that body cells take up abnormally high amounts of glucose and fat, which causes them to produce free radicals and release a host of pro-inflammatory chemicals, such as free radicals, prostaglandins, and cytokines.

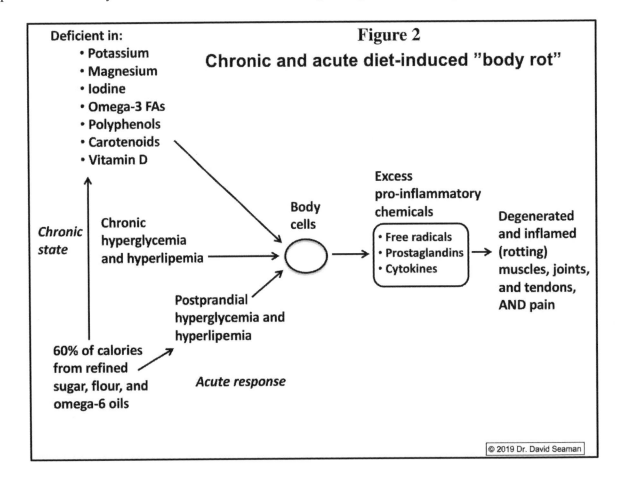

The deceptive issue about eating pro-inflammatory foods is that when we are young and pig out on these foods, they just taste good. There will be a postprandial increase in the cellular production of pro-inflammatory chemicals, but young healthy people who engulf a big dose of refined sugar, flour, and omega-6 oils do not develop painful symptoms because their young tissues have yet to begin the rotting process. The problem is when overeating these refined calories becomes a chronic lifestyle choice, which is the case for most adult Americans and many teenagers. Figure 2 illustrates chronic and acute dietary inflammation.

It is important to understand that refined sugar, flour, and omega-6 oil calories lack vitamins, minerals, anti-inflammatory omega-3 fatty acids, and other nutrients, such as the anti-inflammatory pigments in vegetation, known as polyphenols and carotenoids that give vegetation their characteristic colors. These key nutrients are required to keep the production of pro-inflammatory chemicals in the normal range. Without these key nutrients, the pro-inflammatory chemicals progressively rise to abnormal levels, which can progressively degenerate, inflame, and create a painful rotting state in our muscles, joints, tendons, and spinal discs. Note that many of the key nutrients listed in Figure 2 are taken as nutritional supplements by many people. I will address this topic in Chapter 9.

Consider the following inflammatory scenario that applies to multiple millions of people. In the chronic state, people live 24 hours per day with hyperglycemia and hyperlipemia, which leads to an over production of pro-inflammatory chemicals all day long; a chronic state of body rot. This chronic state is magnified whenever these people eat refined sugar, flour, and oils. These acute and chronic inflammation scenarios are then further magnified because of the lack of key nutrients that are needed to suppress inflammatory activity. The most obvious outcome of this state of chronic inflammatory rotting is chronic pain.

Even worse, this same rotting inflammation state promotes the expression of depression, malaise, and chronic diseases such as heart disease, diabetes, cancer, and Alzheimer's disease. All of these symptoms and diseases prevent one from enjoying their favorite physical activities.

Thus far, I have used basic language when describing the pro-inflammatory chemicals (free radicals, prostaglandins, and cytokines). In Chapter 8, these chemicals will be described in more detail so you can better visualize how The DeFlame Diet can reduce the production of these chemicals back to normal levels to reverse the ongoing state of body rot.

Reference

1. Seaman DR. The diet-induced proinflammatory state: A cause of chronic pain and other degenerative diseases. J Manip Physiol Ther. 2002;25:168-179.
2. Seaman DR. Anti-inflammatory diet for pain patients. Pract Pain Management. 2012;12(10)36-46.
3. Seaman DR. Body mass index and musculoskeletal pain: is there a connection? Chiropractic Man Ther. 2013;21:15.

4. Seaman DR. Weight gain as a consequence of living a modern lifestyle: a discussion of barriers to effective weight control and how to overcome them. J Chiro Humanities. 2013;20(1):27-35.

Chapter 7
Body movement in the context of
diet-induced body rot

Effective and pain-free body movements are difficult to achieve if our muscles, joints, tendons, spinal discs, and bones are rotting due to chronic inflammation. Biomechanics is the scientific term for body movement. The topic is exclusively taught, learned, and conceptualized as if the body is a car, robot, or any other inanimate mechanical device. This mechanical view is taught to most healthcare professionals, including chiropractors, medical doctors, osteopaths, and physical therapists. The perception is that body movement is a mechanical event and injuries to muscles, joints, and tendons are due to excessive mechanical loading, which is a vague term that should be avoided in my opinion. The use of the term "mechanical" directs attention away from the fact that movement is actually a chemical event, which will be described shortly.

There are two types of loading patterns that impact our musculoskeletal tissues. Whether we bend forwards, backwards, sideways or more in rotation, we create compressive (squishing) and tensile (pulling) loads. Both are often referred to as mechanical loading, which, as stated above, is a vague term and not worth using. Compressive loading refers to a force or load that squishes the tissues. Joints, spinal discs, and bones deal with compressive loading. Whenever we pick up an object to carry or workout with, compressive forces are created by the added load (weight of the object) and are absorbed by joints, spinal discs, and bones.

In contrast, tendons do not deal with compressive loading. Tendons attach to both muscle and bone. Whenever a muscle contracts, it pulls on the tendon, which means that tendons deal with tensile (pulling) loads. Again, for the purpose of emphasis, the term "mechanical loading" does not further clarify these two loading patterns that our body chemistry must deal with and worse, only serves to lead one away from understanding that body movements and physical injuries are actually chemical events.

What I am suggesting here is not just an issue of semantics. If we do not view the human body as chemistry, then it is very difficult to conceptualize how musculoskeletal tissues rot and become injury-prone during normal non-injurious compressive and tensile loading events, which is the most common way that musculoskeletal pains emerge.

The human body is made of proteins, fats, carbohydrates, vitamins, minerals, and water. More specifically, we are made of oxygen, carbon, hydrogen, nitrogen, calcium, phosphorus, potassium, magnesium, sodium, sulfur, chloride, and less abundant trace elements like selenium, boron, molybdenum, and others, as well as vitamins. Clearly, the human body is a mass of chemistry, which moves. In other words, biomechanics should be viewed as body chemistry in motion. If this strikes you as odd, consider the fact that approximately 60% of the body is water (1), which consists of hydrogen and oxygen. Muscles are almost 80% water (1), and it is our muscles (sacks of water) that create joint movement. Joint cartilage is 70% water (2), and our bones are 31% water (1). This means that we can almost conceptualize biomechanics as our body water in motion.

Now for a simple question…where do we acquire all of the elements listed in the previous paragraph? We get these elements from breathing, eating anti-inflammatory foods, and drinking water.

Envision that you are a golfer and walking up to the tee to hit a ball. You walk up to the ball while you repeat your swing thoughts…thoughts are neurological chemical events. You tell yourself to take practice strokes that will resemble your actual stroke to hit the ball. Muscle contractions that make the practice swing are directed by the nervous system via a series of chemical events. The generation of a muscle contraction is also a chemical event. When muscles contract they tug on tendons and cause joint movement, which involves the production of chemicals in muscles, tendons, and joints.

With the above movement scenario in mind, which applies to any and all physical activities, it should be obvious that viewing movement as a mechanical event, in the absence of chemistry, is incorrect. It is important that you do not feel foolish if you thought movement was mechanical. I did not realize that biomechanics is actually biochemistry in motion until long after I was taught the inaccurate mechanical dogma of movement. To help shift biomechanical thinking away from "mechanics" to body chemistry in motion, I recently wrote a chapter about this topic in the third edition of a popular book about rehabilitating injuries titled, *Rehabilitation of the spine: a patient-centered approach* (3).

With the above in mind, consider the fact that exercise and physical exertion, as in playing golf, tennis, weight lifting, yard work, etc., involves the production of free radicals, prostaglandins, and cytokines by muscles, joints, and tendons (4-7), which is totally normal and desirable, as they initiate the healing response which is supposed to include a pro-inflammatory response that is followed by an anti-inflammatory response. The same sequence should occur after injuries. If we lack the anti-inflammatory component of the healing process, chronic inflammation and pain will develop. It turns out that a pro-inflammatory diet prevents the anti-inflammatory component of healing, which becomes a 24-hour per day chronic state of body rot for most when they become obese (8).

In summary, body movement is basically our sacks of water (muscles, joints, discs, and bones) sloshing around in a controlled fashion to create compressive and tensile loading patterns, which is dependent on a host of chemical substances, including protein, fat, carbohydrate, vitamins and minerals. Since our bodies are made of chemistry, the chemical choices we make in the form of food will impact how we move and respond to physically and mentally stressful events. Not surprisingly, my suggestion is to eat mostly or exclusively anti-inflammatory foods and avoid refined sugar, flour, and omega-6 oils as outlined in Chapter 1. Being that this is difficult, we should endeavor to reduce our consumption of pro-inflammatory foods to keep the inflammatory markers listed in Chapter 3 in the normal range. This way we allow these objective markers to be our eating guide and not our emotional desires for pro-inflammatory foods.

In the next chapter, I am going to show you how a pro-inflammatory diet causes an over-production of free radicals, prostaglandins, and cytokines, which then leads to physical rotting and chronic pain. If you are still not sure what these chemicals are, it will become clear in Chapter 8.

References:

1. The water in you: water and the human body.
   https://www.usgs.gov/special-topic/water-science-school/science/water-you-water-and-human-body

2. Morrell KC, Hodge WA, Krebs DE, Mann RW. Corroboration of in vivo cartilage pressures with implications for synovial joint tribology and osteoarthritis causation. Proc Nat Acad Sci. 2005;102:14819-24.

3. Seaman DR. Nutritional considerations for inflammation, pain, and rehabilitation. In Liebenson C. Editor. Rehabilitation of the spine: a patient-centered approach. 3rd Edition. New York: Wolters Kluwer; 2019; p.840-853.

4. Lecarpentier Y. Physiological role of free radicals in skeletal muscles. J Appl Physiol. 103:1917-18.

5. Langberg H, Boushel D, Skovgaard D, Risum N, Kjaer M. Cyclo-oxygenase-2 mediated prostaglandin release regulates blood flow in connective tissue during mechanical loading in humans. J Physiol. 2003;551:683-689.

6. Helmark IC, Mikkelsen UR, Børglum J, et al. Exercise increases interleukin-10 levels both intraarticularly and peri-synovially in patients with knee osteoarthritis: a randomized controlled trial. Arthritis Res Ther. 2010;12(4):R126.

7. Pedersen BK, Steensberg A, Schjerling P. Muscle-derived interleukin-6: possible biological effects. J Physiol. 2001;536⊗Pt 2):329-37.

8. Seaman DR. Body mass index and musculoskeletal pain: is there a connection? Chiropractic Man Ther. 2013;21:15.

Chapter 8
Body rot chemistry: Excess free radicals, prostaglandins, and cytokines

This will be the chapter with the most biochemistry, which is unavoidable if you really want to understand how to prevent your body from rotting, so you can be more physically active and have less pain. While Figure 1 likely looks daunting at first glance, it is not difficult to understand, so don't freak out. You may have to read this chapter a few times, which is normal and how learning works.

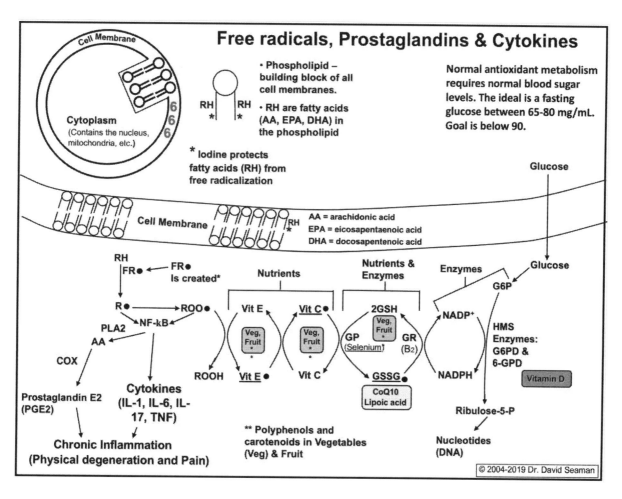

Learning new things can be particularly annoying for adults. I recently transformed my yard into a mini food forest, which took me about two years to complete. I planted dozens of trees, during which time I learned how to improperly and then properly plant and water-in a new tree. I also had to learn the many facets of tree care, insect control, weed control, pruning, and fertilizer use. Many of the words I learned during this process were new to me, but I had to go through the process to become somewhat proficient at managing my transformed yard. I also had to work through the annoyance of dealing with different, and sometimes contradictory, recommendations I received at various nurseries and in the garden section of stores like Lowes and Home Depot.

As I write this book, I am also helping a friend rehab an old house he bought for retirement purposes. I had no idea how many names exist to describe wooden beams in a house (studs, jack stud, king stud, header, joist, ledger board, plates, etc., etc.). It also makes no sense to me why they created the term "flashing" to describe a sheet of metal that protects the roof or wall from water seepage. How about this one; did you know that a soil stack is a plumbing vent pipe that penetrates the roof? The list goes on and on, and my point is that in order to be of help to my friend, I am learning building lingo that I was unfamiliar with. It is actually not so bad, as I want to learn about construction and rehab, but it just takes time and can be frustrating, which is the nature of learning about anything new that is multifaceted in its complexity.

The first thing you need to do is look at the abbreviations in Figure 1. Then look at Table 1 and you will see descriptions for each. Spend a little time familiarizing yourself with the abbreviations and the descriptions. Then only look at the abbreviations and test yourself to see if you can remember the descriptions.

Table 1. Key to Figure 1

Abbreviations	Descriptions
FR•	Free radical
RH	Fatty acid in phospholipid, also called a lipid
R•	Fatty acid radical or lipid radical
ROO•	Lipid peroxyl radical
Vit E•	Vitamin E radical
Vit C•	Vitamin C radical
2GSH	Reduced glutathione (an antioxidant made by the body)
GSSG•	Oxidized or "free radicalized" glutathione
GP	Glutathione peroxidase (antioxidant enzyme that requires selenium)
GR	Glutathione reductase (antioxidant enzyme that requires riboflavin [vitamin B2])
NF-kB	Nuclear Factor-kappa B (key inflammation signaling molecule)
PLA2	Phospholipase A2 (enzyme that clips fatty acids off of phospholipids to promote or reduce inflammation). PLA2 is inhibited by corticosteroids.
COX	Cyclooxygenase (enzyme that converts arachidonic acid [AA] in prostaglandin E2 [PGE2]. COX is inhibited by anti-inflammatory drugs (aspirin, ibuprofen, Tylenol, etc.)
AA	Arachidonic acid (an omega-6 fatty acid found in excess in meat, fish, chicken that was fed a grain-based diet)
EPA	Eicosapentaenoic acid (an omega-3 fatty acid found in fish oil, cold water fish, and any animal that eats green vegetation – such as grass-fed cattle)
DHA	Docosahexaenoic acid (an omega-3 fatty acid found in fish oil, cold water fish, and any animal that eats green vegetation – such as grass-fed cattle)

After you understand this chapter and familiarize yourself with the language and concepts, you will understand how diet causes inflammation at a level higher than most people you know, and will also understand why people become reliant on medications with unwanted side effects (Table 2). In the context of this book, it is important to understand that the daily use of any of these medications means that the body is overtly rotting.

Notice in Table 1 that PLA2 and COX are enzymes that lead to the production of prostaglandin E2 (PGE2). PLA2 clips diet-derived arachidonic acid from a cell membrane phospholipid. When this happens the COX enzyme converts diet-derived arachidonic acid into inflammation and pain-promoting PGE2. This sequence is illustrated in the bottom left side of Figure 1.

Anyone who is taking anti-inflammatory drugs like ibuprofen are doing so to inhibit the COX enzyme to block the production of pain-promoting PGE2. Table 2 lists some of the side effects of the medications used to inhibit PLA2, COX (prostaglandin E2), and the various pro-inflammatory cytokines. This is not a complete list, so if you are interested you can do an internet search for the individual medications. The website rxlist.com is a pharmacy website that provides reliable information.

Table 2. Medications that inhibit inflammatory chemicals

Inflammatory chemicals	Medications	Side-effects
PLA2 (Phospholipase A2)	Corticosteroids (Prednisone, Celestone, Medrol, etc.)	Osteoporosis, hypertension, diabetes, weight gain, increased risk of infections
PGE2 (Prostaglandin E2)	COX inhibiting drugs: aspirin, ibuprofen (Advil), naproxen (Alleve), etc., and Celebrex, and Tylenol	Heartburn, stomach ulcers, high blood pressure, tinnitus, reduced bone healing
IL-1 (interleukin-1)	Kineret	Nausea, vomiting, diarrhea, stomach pain, joint pain, flu symptoms
IL-6 (interleukin-6)	Actemra	Sinus pain, sore throat, headache, dizziness, itching, urinary tract infection
IL-17 (interleukin-17)	Siliq, Taltz, Cosentyx	Joint pain, headache, fatigue, diarrhea, nausea, muscle pain
TNF (Tumor necrosis factor)	Enbrel, Remicade, Humira	Mild nausea, vomiting, diarrhea, headache, stomach pain, heart burn

It is important to understand that these side effects typically occur with long-term use, which can vary from patient to patient. Please consult with your prescribing physician if you have any concerns about these medications, particularly if you have any of these side effects which can be disruptive to life in general, and also quite disruptive to you being able to engage in your favorite physical activities. It is much better to do everything we can to become free of the "flame" so that we do not end up taking these medications.

Note also please that COX inhibiting drugs are typically called non-steroidal anti-inflammatory drugs or NSAIDs. Table 2 lists some of the side effects of these medications. Tylenol is not typically referred to as an NSAID; however, it also functions to inhibit the COX enzyme, so as to reduce the production of painful PGE2. The most common side-effect concern for Tylenol is liver damage, which has the potential to lead to liver failure if Tylenol is regularly taken by people who drinking alcohol.

Back to Figure 1. The first thing that might catch your eye in Figure 1 is the cell in the top left with 666 in the cell membrane. The obvious Biblical reference notwithstanding, the 666 in this case refers to the overconsumption of omega-6 fatty acids that get inserted into cell membranes to create a pro-inflammatory state of body rot. We are supposed to consume a diet of less than a 4 to 1 ratio of omega-6 to omega-3 fatty acids in the diet, which is described in more detail in several chapters in *The DeFlame Diet* book (Chapters 18, 25, 26). To the point of this chapter, an excess of omega-6 oil consumption promotes a state of free radical excess (1), and an over production of PGE2. Ideally, the ratio of omega-6 to omega-3 should be 1:1; which would lead to a 6363 configuration in the cell membrane. This represents an anti-free radical, anti-inflammatory, and a non-painful state, which means an anti-rotting state.

To the right of the cell is a blown-up image of a single phospholipid. An almost countless number of phospholipids are connected together to make up the cell membrane of all cells in the human body. The circle represents what is called the phosphate head and the two vertical lines are fatty acids. It is important to understand that these fatty acids can be omega-6 or omega-3.

The last thing we want is to load up our cell membrane phospholipids with omega-6 fatty acids at the expense of omega-3 fatty acids. The average American eats a 10:1 to 25:1 ratio of omega-6 to omega-3, which is the result of fatty grain-fed animals, and foods cooked/prepared with refined omega-6 oils from corn, sunflower, safflower, cottonseed, peanut, and soybean. The proper omega-6 to omega-3 ratio should be less than 4:1 at worst; ideally as stated above, the ratio should be 1:1. In short, if you overeat omega-6 fatty acids, you will promote a gradual state of body rot in your musculoskeletal tissues.

To the far right in Figure 1, it states that we need proper blood glucose levels in order to promote a proper free radical and antioxidant balance. Too much glucose in the blood supply leads to an excess production of free radicals, which cannot be controlled by dietary antioxidants or our body's antioxidant system.

Our antioxidant system involves both nutrients from our diet and our built-in antioxidant system that involves enzymes (which are a type of protein) that are a normal part of body function. In actual fact, nutrients and enzymes work together to keep free radical production at a healthy and non-rotting level.

The problem that most people have when it comes to understanding antioxidants and free radicals is that they do not understand that supplementation cannot fix the antioxidant enzyme system. In other words, overeating refined sugar, flour, and omega-6 oils creates a perpetual free radical (body rot) state; in part by nutrient deficiency, but also by altering the normal function of our antioxidant enzyme system that favors an excess of free radicals. This means that the most important antioxidant activity we can engage in is the elimination of excess calories from refined sugar, flour, and oils. Consider also that overeating these calories leads to obesity and type 2 diabetes, both of which are body rot inflammatory states that are associated with an excess production of free radicals (2-4), which goes on 24 hours per day in an unrelenting fashion.

It is important to understand that overeating refined sugar, flour, and omega-6 oils creates a rotting state wherein free radicals are perpetually overproduced, which cannot be corrected by supplements. This means we must DeFlame the diet to stop our bodies from rotting.

It is important to understand that free radicals are created constantly in the body by virtue of our dependency on oxygen to survive. Imagine that you bite an apple and let it sit on your counter. Within a short period of time, the flesh exposed to the air by the bite will begin to turn brown. This apple would rapidly rot compared to one sitting next to it on the counter that was not bitten.

The apple browning process is called oxidation, and in the human body, such oxidation refers to free radical production. If you were to take two bites on opposite sides of the apple and squeeze lemon juice on one side, you will notice that it oxidizes much slower compared to the other side. This is because lemons contain antioxidants that prevent oxidation. Our goal with diet and supplements is the same as what the lemon is doing: to keep free radical production at a normal level to prevent our bodies from rotting.

On the far left in Figure 1, you can see that a free radical is created and attacks a fatty acid in the cell membrane to create a lipid radical (R•), which can be converted into a lipid peroxyl radical (ROO•) [remember that lipid is synonymous with fat]. Both of these free radicals can stimulate NF-kB (a key inflammation signaling molecule) to stimulate ongoing inflammation, which manifests as an overproduction of PGE2 and pro-inflammatory cytokines. To the immediate right of these free radicals you can see vitamins E and C, which are specific nutrients that can reduce lipid and lipid peroxyl radicals. This is the extent to which most people think about free radicals and antioxidants, which is a very limited view.

Notice what happens to Vitamin E after it reduces the lipid peroxyl radical…Vitamin E now becomes a free radical. Vitamin C then comes along and reduces the vitamin E radical. But now vitamin C becomes a free radical. For context, adding supplemental vitamins E and C to rotting bodies does little if any good. Rotting bodies lack the antioxidant wherewithal to reduce free radical E and C, which means that radicalized E and C participate in the rotting process. In order for radicalized E and C to be reduced, a substance called reduced glutathione (2GSH) must come to the rescue, which involves both nutrients and enzymes.

As stated above and in Table 1, 2GSH is called reduced glutathione, which is a special antioxidant that our bodies make from three amino acids called cysteine, glycine, and glutamic acid. Then the enzyme glutathione peroxidase, which requires selenium, utilizes 2GSH to reduce the vitamin C radical back to its normal antioxidant vitamin C. But now 2GSH is radicalized into GSSG• and must be reduced back into 2GSH. This requires the enzyme glutathione reductase (GR), which requires riboflavin (vitamin B2) and NADPH. Supplemental lipoic acid and CoQ10 can assist in the process of reducing GSSG• back into 2GSH.

We need proper blood glucose levels to produce NADPH from NADP, which is why maintaining a proper blood glucose level is the most important thing we can do to keep free radical production in the normal range. There are two enzymes (GSPD and 6-GPD) involved in the production of NADPH, which require vitamin D to function properly. NADPH stands for nicotinamide adenine dinucleotide phosphate. Nicotinamide, also referred to as niacinamide, is produced in the body from the B-vitamin niacin. As illustrated in Figure 1, niacinamide-containing NADP+ must be converted into niacinamide-containing NADPH. We must produce adequate levels of NADPH in our bodies, as it is the key antioxidant that supports our body's entire antioxidant system.

Notice in Figure 1 that polyphenols and carotenoids in vegetables and fruit function as antioxidants to help keep vitamin E, vitamin C, and glutathione from becoming free radicalized. Polyphenols and carotenoids are the pigments that give vegetation their characteristic colors. Many people are aware that turmeric and ginger are anti-inflammatory and have antioxidant activity; it is the polyphenols in these spices that are responsible for these beneficial functions.

Note also in Figure 1, that iodine protects fatty acids from being radicalized (5). This is a mostly unknown fact, which is why we should make sure to ingest adequate amounts of iodine or take an iodine supplement. Seaweed and fish are the best dietary sources of iodine. Supplemental iodine will be discussed in Chapter 9.

The end result of an excess of free radical generation is the overproduction of prostaglandin E2 (PGE2) and the proinflammatory cytokines as illustrated in the bottom left of Figure 1. When PGE2 and pro-inflammatory cytokines are overproduced during the majority of a lifespan, they participate in the gradual rotting or degradation of muscles, joints, tendons, spinal discs and bones (6-17), which of course, is a disaster for people who wish to remain physically active. The rotting process of each tissue will be discussed in separate chapters in this book.

In the next chapter, I will discuss supplementing with key nutrients that have been mentioned in this current chapter and previously in Chapter 6. My approach to supplementation is to focus on the key nutrients that have the biggest effect on helping to control inflammation.

References

1. Berry EM. Are diets high in omega-6 polyunsaturated fatty acids unhealthy? Eur Heart J Suppl. 2001;3(Supplement D):D37-D41.
2. Hakkak R, Korourian S, Melnyk S. Obesity, oxidative stress and breast cancer risk. J Cancer Sci Ther. 2013;5(12):1000e129.
3. Kruk J. Overweight, obesity, oxidative stress and the risk of breast cancer. Asian Pac J Cancer Prev. 2014;15:9579-86.
4. Ullah A, Khan A, Khan I. Diabetes mellitus and oxidative stress—a concise review. Saudi Pharmaceutical J. 2016;24:547-553.
5. Venturi S, Venturi M. Iodine, PUFAs and iodolipids in health and diseases: an evolutionary perspective. 2014;29:185-205.
6. Dalle S, Rossmeislova L, Koppo K. The role of inflammation in age-related sarcopenia. Front Physiol. 2017;8: Article 1045.
7. Fan J, Kou X, Yang Y, Chen N. MicroRNA-regulated proinflammatory cytokines in sarcopenia. Mediators Inflammation. 2016; Article ID 1428686.
8. Bonnet CS, Walsh DA. Osteoarthritis, angiogenesis and inflammation. Rheumatol. 2005;44:7-16.
9. Dakin SG, Dudhia J, Smith RK. Resolving an inflammatory concept. The importance of inflammation and resolution in tendinopathy. Vet Immunol Immunopathol. 2014;158(3-4):121-27.
10. Millar NL, Murrell GA, McInnes IB. Inflammatory mechanisms in tendinopathy – towards translation. Nat Rev Rheumatol. 2017;13:110-22.
11. Grange L, Gaudin P, Trocme C, et al. Intervertebral disk degeneration and herniation: the role of metalloproteinases and cytokines. Joint Bone Spine. 2001;68:547-53.
12. Risbud MV, Shapiro IM. Role of cytokines in intervertebral disc degeneration: pain and disc-content. Nat Rev Rheumatol. 2014;10:44-56.
13. Weber KT, Alipui DO, Sison CP, et al. Serum levels of the proinflammatory cytokine interleukin-6 vary based on diagnoses in individuals with lumbar intervertebral disc diseases. Arthritis Res Ther. 2016;18:3.
14. Sadowska A, Touli E, Hitzl W, et al. Inflammaging in cervical and lumbar degenerated intervertebral discs: analysis of proinflammatory cytokine and TRP channel expression. Eur Spine J. 2018;27:564-77.
15. Sadowska A, Hausmann ON, Wuertz-Kozak K. Inflammaging in the intervertebral disc. Clin Trans Neurosci. 2018;Jan-June:1-9.
16. Lencel P, Magne D. Inflammaging: the driving force in osteoporosis? Med Hypothesis. 2011;76:317-21.
17. Pietschmann P, Mechtcheriakova D, Mechtcheriakova A, Foger-Samwald U, Ellinger I. Immunology of osteoporosis: a mini-review. Gerontology. 2016;62:128-37.

Chapter 9
Supplements to reduce inflammation

In the previous chapter about free radicals and inflammation, multiple nutrients were discussed. Naturally this leads to the question as to whether they should be taken as supplements. This chapter addresses that question.

It is quite common for people to misunderstand the purpose of nutritional supplements. They are typically viewed in the context of taking medications, which is also viewed in a fashion that is inaccurate. Here is what I mean. A pro-inflammatory lifestyle, which includes a poor diet, stress, a lack of sleep, and sedentary living, cause our bodies to literally rot (chronic inflammation) and then express disease. While certain drugs and supplements can be helpful, it is impossible for them to correct lifestyle-induced body rot. Below is Figure 2 from Chapter 6.

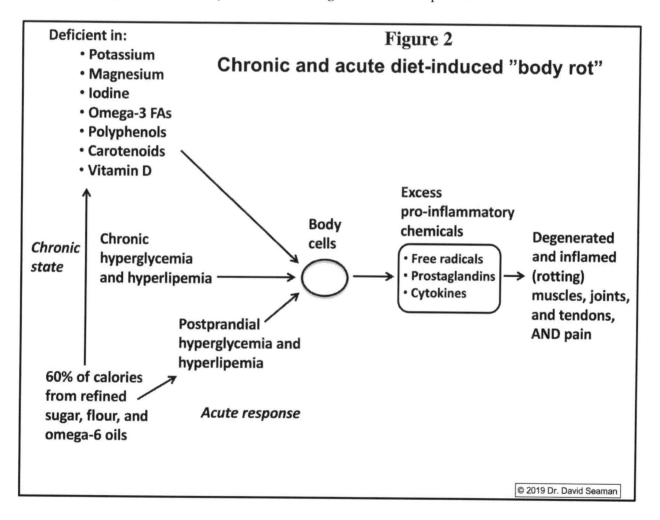

Approximately 70% of the US population is overweight or obese, which represents a state of chronic inflammation. In other words, 70% of our population is literally rotting.

The average American eats far too many calories, of which approximately 60% are derived from refined sugar, flour, and omega-6 oils. This leads to gradual weight gain, which is accompanied by deficiencies of the key nutrients listed in Figure 2. As stated above, when this diet-induced pro-inflammatory state manifests itself, no drug or combination of drugs can remotely restore a normal state of non-inflammatory chemistry to the body. The same holds true for supplements, which is why it is so important to achieve and maintain a body weight that allows for the markers of inflammation outlined in Chapter 3 to return to normal. In most cases, when the markers of inflammation are normal, people can live most of their lives without medications. However, this does not necessarily mean we should avoid taking key supplements.

Many people believe that if you eat properly, you do not need to take any supplements. I disagree with this view. My perspective is that we should all take certain supplements, those being magnesium, iodine, omega-3 fatty acids, polyphenols, and vitamin D, which are listed in Figure 2.

Notice that potassium is NOT recommended as a supplement. We should get potassium exclusively from food because it is released slowly during the digestive process. This prevents a rapid rise in blood potassium levels, which can otherwise happen for some people if they take potassium supplements. A high potassium level is called hyperkalemia, which can lead to heart rhythm changes, called arrhythmias. The person most likely to suffer from a fatal arrhythmia is someone who has diabetes, chronic kidney disease, and is also taking certain blood pressure medications called angiotensin converting enzyme (ACE) inhibitors or angiotensin receptor blockers (ARB). To read more about this topic and to see a full list of conditions and medications that cause hyperkalemia, you can do an internet search for the following article:

Hollander-Rodriguez JC, Calvert JF. Hyperkalemia. Am Fam Phys. 2006;73(2):283-90.

It would be especially advisable to consult with your physician if you fall into the category of the person described in the previous paragraph or are taking medications that elevate blood potassium levels. More details about the anti-inflammatory nature of potassium can be found in *The DeFlame Diet* book.

Compared to potassium, there is typically no problem with taking the nutrients listed above in Figure 2. Nonetheless, it is always advisable to consult with your physician to identify potential drug/nutrient interactions.

What follows is my view of the utility of supplements. I am purely interested in the DeFlaming outcome of supplements; a view that I would urge you to consider adopting. The supplements will be discussed in the order they appear in Figure 1. I do not believe we need to take carotenoid supplements. Carotenoids are packed into all vegetables, especially leafy green vegetables.

Magnesium

There are more than 300 metabolic reactions in the body that require magnesium, and many involve anti-inflammatory actions. The typical recommendation for magnesium supplementation is 400-1000 mg per day. I personally take at least 1000 mg per day. I often take more if I am feeling especially stressed out because stress physiology depletes body magnesium (1).

Iodine

Iodine is most known for its relationship to the production of thyroid hormones. Not well known is what was described in the previous chapter about iodine; that it functions as an antioxidant and protects cell membrane fatty acids from free radical attack. This is important for all cell membranes; however, in the context of disease risk, it is especially important for protection against breast cancer and prostate cancer (2,3). The Japanese population consumes between 1000-3000 micrograms (mcg) per day (2), which is derived largely from seaweed and much less from fish. It turns out that seaweed and fish are natural sources of both omega-3 fatty acids and iodine, which is one of the reasons why a traditional Japanese diet is so healthy and associated with minimal disease risk. When Japanese people move to the United States and adopt a pro-inflammatory American diet, they begin to express the same chronic diseases as Americans.

In the United States, the upper limit recommendation for iodine is only 1100 mcg per day. I personally take 1000 mcg per day in addition to my diet, which means I choose to ingest iodine based on the Japanese intake pattern. As far as I can tell, the 1000-3000 mcg level is likely to be a problem for only people with hypothyroidism caused by Hashimoto's disease (2). Many people with Hashimoto's disease cannot take any iodine. If you consider taking iodine, consult with your physician if you have concerns about hypothyroidism caused by Hashimoto's disease.

Omega-3 fatty acids

Supplementing with omega-3 fatty acids from fish oil is quite common and many people do it. The typical recommendation is to take between 1000-3000 milligrams (mg) per day. The purpose of taking omega-3 fatty acids is to create a proper balance of omega-6 to omega-3 fatty acids in our cell membranes, which was discussed in the previous chapter. Recall that most Americans consume a 10:1 to 25:1 ratio of omega-6 to omega-3 fatty acids. There are two mistakes that people make when they supplement with omega-3 fish oil.

The first mistake most people make is to take omega-3 fish oil supplements without simultaneously eliminating the excess omega-6 oils. As stated previously, omega-6 fatty acids are found in great abundance in oils from corn, safflower, sunflower, cottonseed, peanut, and soybean oils. The most notable caloric culprits that are rich in omega-6 fatty acids include cakes, desserts, donuts, French fries (and other deep-fried foods), and oil roasted nuts. Additionally, all feed lot-raised animals (meat, fish, chicken) have an abundance of omega-6 fatty acids compared to their natural counterparts as a consequence of the excess omega-6 fatty acids in the feed.

The second mistake is to not recognize that omega-3 rich foods in nature are also the best sources of omega-3 fatty acid-protecting iodine. Seaweed is particularly abundant, while fish is less and fish oil contains virtually no iodine due to the distillation process involved in making fish oil supplements.

As my knowledge about iodine has expanded, I now believe it is foolish to take omega-3 fish oil supplements without also ensuring adequate iodine intake as outlined in the previous section about iodine.

Polyphenols

As described in the previous chapter, polyphenols and carotenoids are found in vegetation. I never supplement with carotenoids because I eat lots of green vegetables, which are a rich source. I do supplement ginger and/or turmeric to increase my intake of polyphenols. I also often take polyphenols derived from lemons. The typical recommendation is about 1000-2000 milligrams per day of supplemental polyphenols. When I make fresh vegetable juice, I always use ginger and/or turmeric as well as lemons and/or limes.

Vitamin D

Vitamin D supplementation has become very popular in recent years. I typically take about 5000 IUs per day. Important to understand is that I do this for the purpose of maintaining an adequate vitamin D level, which is anti-inflammatory. I will discuss vitamin D more in Chapter 11.

Additional supplements

I also take coenzyme Q10 (100 mg/day), glucosamine sulfate (1500 mg/day), and cycle on and off with probiotics, as an anti-inflammatory diet naturally supports a healthy gut flora. Understand again that all of these supplements I take are for the purpose of inflammation reduction and not for the purpose of targeting a specific condition. The various names of conditions and diseases is not relevant when you understand that all chronic conditions are driven by the same underlying pro-inflammatory state.

References
1. Seaman DR. The DeFlame Diet: deflame your diet, body, and mind.
2. Seaman DR. The DeFlame Diet for Breast Health and Cancer Prevention.
3. Venturi S, Venturi M. Iodine, PUFAs and iodolipids in health and diseases: an evolutionary perspective. 2014;29:185-205.

Chapter 10
Obesity and how it rots the body

Approximately 70% of the adult population in the United States are overweight or obese. The CDC (Centers for Disease Control) in Atlanta indicates that the prevalence of obesity was 35.7% among young adults aged 20 to 39 years, 42.8% among middle-aged adults aged 40 to 59 years, and 41.0% among older adults aged 60 and older. In the under 20 age group, almost 20% are obese. Clearly, obesity has reached epidemic proportions.

People still misunderstand obesity to be merely a condition of excess calorie storage. In fact, obesity is a chronic inflammatory state of body rot that promotes all chronic diseases, including diabetes, Alzheimer's disease, heart disease, cancer, AND germane to this book, chronic pain and musculoskeletal degeneration. Clearly, avoiding obesity is very important for people who are physically active.

First, as stated in previous chapters, as we age, we naturally flame up; this is the case for everyone. Dying of old age is the ultimate inflammatory event – no specific chronic disease is required. We cannot live forever, even if we are physically active, lean, fit, and free of disease. The goal should be to *not* exaggerate and accelerate the inflammaging process to the point of body rot, which is why obesity is such a problem.

Obesity is always associated with an uptick in inflammation to enhance overall body rot; however, this is less severe when we are young and becomes progressively more severe as we inflammage. Additionally, in most cases, older obese individuals have typically been obese and rotting for many decades, which means that they have lived with the chronic inflammatory state of obesity for an extended number of years while they were simultaneously inflammaging.

What is it about obesity that is promotional for musculoskeletal degeneration and pain? Part of the problem is elevated blood glucose levels and related problems, which will be the focus of Chapter 12. In the present chapter, we are going to focus on pro-inflammatory biochemistry that exists in excess body fat that serves to "flame up" and rot the entire body, including our musculoskeletal tissues. Body fat, also called adipose tissue, is made up of two primary cell types, those being fat cells and immune cells, which together create the adipose organ.

Fat cells (adipocytes)
Fat cells, also called adipocytes, produce two important hormones that will be discussed in this section, those being adiponectin and leptin. Because these hormones are secreted by adipocytes, they are collectively referred to as adipokines or adipocytokines. Each will be discussed below.

Adiponectin

Adiponectin production levels by fat cells are directly related to adiposity, which means the degree of body fatness. Fat cells can either be lean, overweight, or obese, or in transition among one of these three states. Lean fat cells produce proper amounts of adiponectin, which is then released into body circulation to deliver multiple anti-inflammatory functions. As body fatness increases, there is a commensurate reduction in adiponectin production, and therefore, less adiponectin in circulation and less anti-inflammatory activity throughout the body. Here is a list of the anti-inflammatory effects (anti-rotting effects) of adiponectin that are lost as one progresses toward the chronic inflammatory state of obesity (1):

Skeletal muscle: adiponectin increases fat burning (properly called fat oxidation for energy production), increases skeletal muscle response to insulin

Liver: adiponectin reduces inflammation, reduces fibrosis, reduces fat infiltration, reduces the production of glucose

Fat cells: adiponectin increases glucose uptake, which helps to maintain normal blood glucose levels

Brain: adiponectin increases energy expenditure, reduces body weight

Macrophages (a specific immune cell): adiponectin reduces foam cell formation, which prevents vascular disease called atherosclerosis

Heart: adiponectin helps to maintain vascular regulation to prevent ischemic injury, which means injury due to reduced blood flow

Endothelial cells (the cells that line all blood vessel walls, which is 60-100 thousand miles of blood vessels inside the human body): adiponectin increases vasodilation (vessel relaxation to improve blood supply to vital organs), reduces adhesion molecules (substances that cause immune cells to stick to each other and to vessel walls)

Smooth muscle cells (the muscles in blood vessel walls that contract/relax and promote atherosclerosis when chronic inflammation is present): adiponectin reduces smooth muscle proliferation and migration, which means adiponectin prevents atherosclerosis

Pancreas: adiponectin protects insulin-producing cells from injury by pro-inflammatory cytokines

All of the above anti-rotting functions are desirable for anyone wishing to maintain normal body function. Consider again please the effect that adiponectin has on skeletal muscle; it increases fat burning and makes muscles more sensitive to insulin. There is one more beneficial effect to consider, which involves mitochondria, the producers of our body's source of energy called adenosine triphosphate or ATP. It turns out that adiponectin increases the number mitochondria in skeletal muscle and improves their ATP-producing function (2). Without adiponectin, the ability of muscle mitochondria to "burn" fat for energy is compromised (3). This means that if you want to keep your muscles functioning properly, you need an adequate supply of adiponectin from healthy, non-obese fat cells.

It is important for me to emphasize, and for you to understand, that adiponectin is only released in proper amounts by non-obese and therefore, non-inflamed fat cells. And because fat cell-derived adiponectin improves the function of multiple organs, especially skeletal muscles in the context of this book, you can see why it is so erroneous to view fat cells as just a place where excess calories are stored. If your fat cells are non-obese, they will help DeFlame your skeletal muscles...quite amazing. However, if our fat mass increases, particularly our abdominal fat mass, all of the beneficial functions of adiponectin are lost to varying degrees, and no drug or nutritional supplement can correct these multiple deficits.

There are two final points about adiponectin for you to think about. First, adiponectin levels in the blood supply are supposed to be 1000-fold higher compared to many pro-inflammatory growth factors and cytokines (4), which is likely how it is able to participate in so many important anti-inflammatory functions. Second, adiponectin also appears to be a systemic (full body/most cells) down-regulator of NF-kB (4), which is a key signaling molecule that causes cells to release prostaglandin E2 and the pro-inflammatory cytokines.

The only way to maintain or restore normal adiponectin levels is to achieve a normal lean body weight. As stated in the first sentence of this chapter, approximately 70% of the adult population is overweight or obese, which means that most of the US population has compromised adiponectin levels.

Leptin
Leptin is the other hormone produced almost exclusively by fat cells (adipocytes). In contrast to adiponectin, which is reduced by obesity, leptin release is increased, such that obese people are described to have hyperleptinemia, which means abnormally elevated blood levels of leptin.

The most well-known function of leptin involves satiation after a meal; that is, you no longer feel hungry. In non-obese individuals, leptin release by fat cells increases after a meal. Leptin travels through the vascular system and reaches the brain, where it stimulates the hypothalamus so that you no longer feel hungry. This function of leptin is gradually lost as the chronic inflammation of obesity progressively increases, such that the inflamed hypothalamus becomes resistant to the satiating effect of leptin, which is called leptin resistance (5,6). The outcome of this is that obese people can still feel hungry even though the gut feels absolutely full and is stuffed with food. This is also why obese people often feel hungry to the point of starving all the time, which causes them to become obsessed with food.

The problem with hyperleptinemia is not limited to feelings of starvation. Too much leptin in circulation compromises skeletal muscle function and promotes disc degeneration and herniation.

When leptin is released in normal amounts from lean healthy fat cells, it (along with adiponectin) supports mitochondria energy production and fat burning. When this function is lost, fat can accumulate in skeletal muscle, which is called "lipotoxicity" (7). Rotting lipotoxic muscles and painful spinal discs will also not help you enjoy your favorite physical activity.

It turns out that hyperleptinemia can augment the inflammation that causes discs to degenerate and herniate (8). This is because leptin potentiates the local production of cytokines and can stimulate the production of disc degrading metalloproteinase enzymes (8).

Body fat immune cells

One of the first studies that identified immune cells in adipose tissue was published in 2003 (9). This is an extremely new finding in science and has changed the way we look at body fatness. Historically, overweight or obese individuals were merely viewed as carriers of excess stored calories. Now we know that adipose tissue is an organ, comprised of two major cell types, those being adipocytes (fat cells) and immune cells, each of which produces numerous chemicals that influence local adipose tissue physiology and systemic (full body and body) physiology.

When we are young and lean, which historically was the case for almost all adolescents, both fat and immune cells release anti-inflammatory chemicals into body circulation. As we age and become stressed out and sedentary overeaters, we start to pack on the fat pounds and this causes both fat and immune cells to release pro-inflammatory chemicals into body circulation that participate in promoting all of the well-known chronic diseases, such as diabetes, osteoarthritis, heart disease, and cancer (10). The transformation of lean adipose tissue that contains healthy anti-inflammatory fat cells and immune cells to obese adipose tissue with pro-inflammatory fat cells and immune cells is called "adipose tissue remodeling" (11).

It is important to understand that the immune cell profile in obese remodeled adipose tissue resembles that of an infection or autoimmune disease. I personally think we should view obesity as a state of being "infected" by excess calories, to which the immune system responds accordingly by releasing a host of pro-inflammatory chemicals, which would otherwise be released only if there is an actual microbial or viral infection. Scientists, in the laboratory setting, have demonstrated that this sentiment is true.

A point of clarification before continuing…it is a mistake to think that our stored fat comes mostly from the fat we eat. In fact, the majority of calories we eat come from refined sugar and flour, which makes up approximately 40% of all the calories Americans consume. The excess sugar/flour calories we eat is converted into *saturated* fat and stored in adipocytes. This means that obese fat cells are packed with stored saturated fat, which mostly comes from overeating refined sugar and flour. For more information about saturated fat, unsaturated fat, trans fat, and cholesterol, check out *The DeFlame Diet* book that contains 60 pages about these topics.

There are two key immune-activating events that occur as adipocytes fill up with fat. One involves a reduction in oxygen levels within the adipose tissue mass, referred to as hypoxia. The hypoxia causes adipocytes to release chemotactic agents, which attract immune cells to enter the hypoxic fat mass (11,12). As obese fat cells age, they become necrotic (cell death) and literally go through a rotting process. These rotting fat cells release their great abundance of stored saturated fatty acids. It turns out that the receptor for microbial antigens (infective proteins) on immune cells, called a Toll-like receptor-4 (TLR4), also responds to the saturated fatty acids that are released by rotting fat cells (12). This means that non-microbial factors are capable of activating the immune system to behave like a chronic low-grade infection is present – in the case of the majority of Americans, we become chronically "infected," not by viruses or bacteria, but by excess calories from sugar, flour, and refined oils. This is why obese people feel unwell, and this is obviously problematic if you want to engage in physical activities.

One of the immune cells found in obese adipose tissue is called a macrophage, whose function is to engulf microbes; however, there are no microbes in body fat. The macrophages show up in abundance to engulf the fat-laden and rotting adipocytes, as if they were microbes. In fact, 90% of the macrophages that enter obese adipose tissue are there to deal with the rotting fat cell (13).

Scientists have examined the structural relationship between necrotic fat cells and macrophages, which is referred to as a crown-like structure (13). Figure 1 on the next page, which is nicely colorized in the Kindle version of this book, illustrates the difference in cell types that make up lean adipose tissue and obese adipose tissue (14-17). Notice how fat cells swell in size as they take in calories and become obese. Also notice how the immune cell population completely changes when lean fat cells are transformed into obese fat cells, and M1 macrophages encircle the necrotic fat cell to create what looks like a crown.

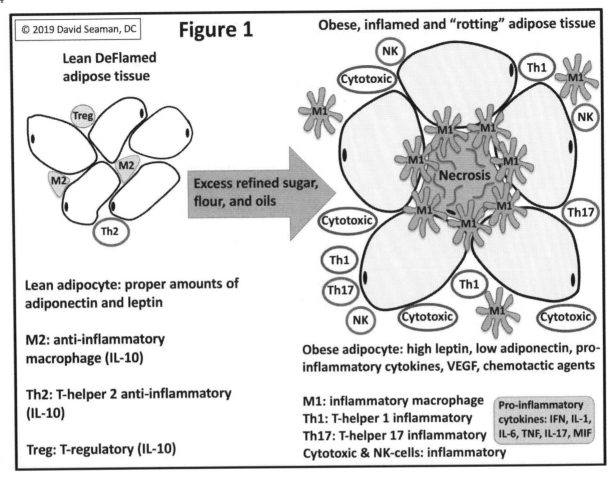

© 2019 David Seaman, DC

Figure 1

Lean DeFlamed adipose tissue

Obese, inflamed and "rotting" adipose tissue

Excess refined sugar, flour, and oils

Necrosis

Lean adipocyte: proper amounts of adiponectin and leptin

M2: anti-inflammatory macrophage (IL-10)

Th2: T-helper 2 anti-inflammatory (IL-10)

Treg: T-regulatory (IL-10)

Obese adipocyte: high leptin, low adiponectin, pro-inflammatory cytokines, VEGF, chemotactic agents

M1: inflammatory macrophage
Th1: T-helper 1 inflammatory
Th17: T-helper 17 inflammatory
Cytotoxic & NK-cells: inflammatory

Pro-inflammatory cytokines: IFN, IL-1, IL-6, TNF, IL-17, MIF

Recall from earlier that lean adipocytes produce the anti-inflammatory adiponectin that circulates at 1000 times the level of pro-inflammatory growth factors and cytokines (IL-1, IL-6, IL-17, TNF, etc.). Lean adipocytes progressively lose the ability to produce adiponectin as they become increasingly more obese, which eventually leads to a depressed level of adiponectin in body circulation, which is highly inflammatory. In contrast, obese adipocytes do not lose their ability to release leptin; in fact, leptin levels in circulation significantly increase, which was discussed earlier in this chapter.

Notice also in Figure 1 that lean adipose tissue contains at least three different anti-inflammatory immune cells, all of which release an extremely important anti-inflammatory cytokine called interleukin-10 (IL-10). The anti-inflammatory macrophage is designated as M2. The other two cells are anti-inflammatory T lymphocytes. One is called a T-helper 2 cell (Th2). The second is a T-regulatory cell (Treg), which releases anti-inflammatory IL-10 and also functions to promote self-tolerance, which means they prevent autoimmune disease expression. Clearly, we all need to have lean anti-inflammatory adipose tissue. Unfortunately, during the obesity process, anti-inflammatory fat cells and immune cells are replaced by those that are pro-inflammatory and capable of perpetually releasing pro-inflammatory chemistry 24 hours per day, which is augmented whenever excess calories are consumed.

The obese adipose tissue illustrated in Figure 1 should scare you…it scares me for sure. Life is difficult enough on so many levels for the average person that no one should self-impose an additional layer of misery on themselves by moving through life with rotting fat cells in their bodies.

Th1 cells (T-helper 1 cells) typically participate in autoimmune disease expression, rheumatoid arthritis and psoriasis being the most well-known. Th1 cells release a cytokine called interferon (IFN) which causes neighboring immune cells, particularly M1 macrophages to release their pro-inflammatory cytokines (IL-1, IL-6, TNF). When IFN was used to treat patients with chronic active hepatitis C, 40% of subjects developed full-blown major depression (18).

Th17 (T-helper 17 cells) were discovered more recently compared to Th1 and Th2 cells. They were named based on their release of interleukin-17 (IL-17), another pro-inflammatory cytokine. The main role of IL-17 in humans is to combat bacterial and fungal infections (19); however, Th-17 cells rapidly accumulate in obese adipose tissue (16), which as stated above is "infected" with excess calories and not microorganisms. IL-17 production is involved in the expression of multiple chronic diseases (16), including joint inflammation (20) and disc herniation (21).

Cytotoxic T-cells and natural killer (NK) cells typically show up to release pro-inflammatory cytokines to combat cancer and viral infections. This information should again alert you to the fact that the human body perceives obesity as a biochemical state that resembles an autoimmune disease, an infection, and/or cancer. No one should be surprised why obese individuals with rotting fat cells are far more likely to be fatigued, lethargic, depressed, and in physical pain compared to their lean counterparts.

The pro-inflammatory transformation illustrated in Figure 1 occurs anywhere that obese fat cells become hypoxic and necrotic. Unfortunately, the average American (70% of us) is either overweight or obese, which means that most Americans are literally rotting to death. Stated in a more scientific way, this means that adipose tissue is remodeled to varying degrees in all of these individuals and resembles, to varying degrees, the pro-inflammatory adipose tissue image in Figure 1. In this state, obese adipose tissue perpetually releases pro-inflammatory cytokines into body circulation by which they promote inflammation in visceral organs and musculoskeletal tissues, causing these tissues to literally rot.

Endotoxin and obesity

Endotoxin is a component of the outer cell wall in gram-negative bacteria. Gram-negative bacteria make up about half the population of bacteria in our digestive tract. Humans have a small amount of endotoxin in body circulation that is derived from the digestive tract. When endotoxin is absorbed it is processed by healthy LDL and HDL cholesterol, which keeps circulating endotoxin at a minimal and clinically irrelevant level. This all changes when we overeat refined sugar, flour, and oil calories and become obese. Endotoxin levels increase above normal, which is called low-grade endotoxemia, a known promoter of chronic inflammation. Any human cell that is impacted by excess circulating endotoxin will respond by releasing cytokines and other pro-inflammatory chemicals. There are essentially three stages by which endotoxin levels rise, which I described in *The DeFlame Diet* book, which add to ongoing body rot.

> First, when we overeat refined sugar, flour, and oil calories, there is a greater release of endotoxin from the bacterial cell wall in our digestive tract, which is then absorbed into body circulation. This happens no matter if you are healthy or sick.

> Second, as people continue to overeat pro-inflammatory calories, the digestive tract flames up and becomes more permeable, which allows for a greater amount of endotoxin to enter body circulation.

> Third, as body fat accumulates, people become obese and develop the pro-inflammatory metabolic syndrome (see Chapter 12 for more details). The metabolic syndrome is a pro-inflammatory state that includes the transformation of healthy LDL and HDL into pro-inflammatory LDL and HDL (see Chapter 13 for more details). When this happens, the inflamed LDL and HDL can no longer properly process and eliminate endotoxin.

In addition to the gut, endotoxin can also get into circulation from our mouths. People with gingivitis, but especially periodontitis, are likely to have an increased level of circulating endotoxin (22). Elevated endotoxin levels have been correlated to many conditions, such as obesity, the metabolic syndrome, diabetes, atherosclerosis, and others, which I outlined in *The DeFlame Diet* book. Later in this book, you will see how endotoxin participates in the degeneration and rotting of musculoskeletal tissues. Additionally, because low-grade endotoxemia promotes chronic systemic inflammation, any condition caused by chronic inflammation can be made worse.

Endotoxin levels can return to normal if people DeFlame their diets and become physically active. Endotoxin is never measured in clinical practice. However, endotoxin levels are measured in the research setting and are known to correlate with other inflammatory markers. So, if you normalize all the inflammatory markers discussed in Chapter 3, endotoxin levels typically normalize as well.

Steps to take to get obesity under control
Many people do not realize how overweight or obese they actually are. My suggestion is to do an internet search for "BMI NIH," which will take you the NIH's website where you can insert your height and weight. Your goal is to be below 25. Next, you want to check your waist/hip ratio and make sure, if you are a woman, yours is below .8 and if you are a man, yours is below .95. If you want to be more detailed in you inflammation tracking, my suggestion is to get *The DeFlame Diet* book and make sure to get all of the inflammatory markers to normal levels.

You should also read *Weight Loss Secrets You Need To Know*, which outlines how to mentally get control of your eating, which is commonly called mindfulness. All the key barriers and challenges to effective weight management are presented in a fashion that will allow you to become the master of your eating environment.

It is not just important to control your caloric intake in general and to specifically eliminate calories from refined sugar, flour, and oil. You also need to dramatically increase your consumption of vegetation, which are loaded with vitamins, minerals, and anti-inflammatory pigments called polyphenols/carotenoids (see the chapter on polyphenols/carotenoids in *The DeFlame Diet* book for more information).

Not surprisingly, exercise is very important for weight management; however, there is a better way to view exercise…it is an extremely anti-inflammatory activity so long as you exercise within your individual tolerance zone. Too little exercise is not enough for DeFlaming purposes, and too much can be pro-inflammatory.

Consider, for example, that exercise training reduces the expression of TLR4 (the Toll-like receptor described above) on immune cells, which helps to down-regulate the inflammatory state (23). Exercise also reduces oxidative stress (excess free radical production) and improves mitochondrial function so that fats and ketones can be readily used as energy (23).

Exercise also increases the body's production of IL-10, the powerful anti-inflammatory cytokine described earlier, and reduces immune cell production of TNF (23). There is also evidence from an obese animal model that exercise can promote the switch from a pro-inflammatory M1 macrophage population to the anti-inflammatory M2 macrophage in adipose tissue (24). Clearly, we should all be engaged in regular exercise.

References

1. Xu A, Wang Y, Lam KS. Adiponectin. In: Fantuzzi G, Mazzone T, Eds. Adipose tissue and adipokines in health and disease. Totowa, NJ: Human Press; 2007: p.47-59.
2. Civitarese AE, Ukropcova B, Carling S, et al. Role of adiponectin in human skeletal muscle bioenergetics. Cell Metab. 2006;4:75-87.
3. Yoon MJ, Lee GY, Chung JJ, et al. Adiponectin increases fatty acid oxidation in skeletal muscle cells by sequential activation of AMP-activated protein kinase, p38 mitogen-activated protein kinase, and peroxisome proliferator-activated receptor alpha. Diabetes. 2006;55:2562-70.
4. Ouchi N, Walsh K. A novel role for adiponectin in the regulation of inflammation. Arterioscler Thromb Vasc Biol. 2008;28:1219-21.
5. Thaler JP, Schwartz MW. Minireview: inflammation and obesity pathogenesis: the hypothalamus heats up. Endocrinol. 2010;151:4109-15.
6. Wisse BE, Schwartz MW. Does hypothalamic inflammation cause obesity? Cell Metab. 2009;10:241-242.
7. Ceddia RB. Direct metabolic regulation in skeletal muscle and fat tissue by leptin: implications for glucose and fatty acids homeostasis. Int J Obes. 2005;29:1175-83.

8. Segar AH, Fairbank JC, Urban J. Leptin and the intervertebral disc: a biochemical link exists between obesity, intervertebral disc degeneration and low back pain—an in vitro study in a bovine model. European Spine J. 2019;28:214-23.

9. Weisberg SP, McCann D, Desai M, et al. Obesity is associated with macrophage accumulation in adipose tissue. J Clin Invest. 2003;112:1796-1808.

10. Seaman DR. Body mass index and musculoskeletal pain: is there a connection? Chiro Man Ther. 2013;21:15.

11. Sun K, Kusminski CM, Scherer PE. Adipose tissue remodeling and obesity. J Clin Invest. 2011;121:2094-2101.

12. Ferrante AW. The immune cells in adipose tissue. Diabetes Obes Meta. 2013;15:34-38.

13. Murano I, Barbatelli G, Parisani V, et al. Dead adipocytes, detected as crown-like structures, are prevalent in visceral fat depots of genetically obese mice. J Lipid Res. 2008;49:1562-68.

14. Harford KA, Reynolds CM, McGillicuddy FC, Roche HM. Fats, inflammation and insulin resistance: insights to the role of macrophage and T-cell accumulation. In adipose tissue. Proc Nutr Soc. 2011;70:408-17.

15. Cautivo KM, Molofsky AB. Regulation of metabolic health and adipose tissue function by group 2 innate lymphoid cells. Eur J Immunol. 2016;46:1315-25.

16. Chehimi M, Vidal H, Eljaafari A. Pathogenic role of IL-17-producing immune cells in obesity, and related inflammatory disease. J Clin Med. 2017;6:68.

17. Reilly SM, Saltiel AR. Adapting to obesity with adipose tissue inflammation. Nat Rev Endocrinol. 2017;13:633-43.

18. Bonaccorso S, Meltzer H, Maees M. Psychological and behavioral effects of interferons. Curr Opin Psychiatry. 2000;13:673-677.

19. Yang B, Kang H, Fung A, et al. The role of interleukin-17 in tumour proliferation, angiogenesis, and metastasis. Mediators Inflamm. 2014:623759.

20. Onishi RM, Gaffen SL. Interleukin-17 and its target genes: mechanisms of interleukin-17 function in disease. Immunology. 2010;129:311-21.

21. Shamji MF, Setton LA, Jarvis W, et al. Proinflammatory cytokine expression profile degenerated and herniated human intervertebral disc tissues. Arthritis Rheum. 2010;62:1974-82.

22. Bui FQ, Almeida-da-Silva CL, Huynh B, et al. Association between periodontal pathogens and systemic disease. Biomed J. 2019;42:27-35.

23. Kruger K. Inflammation during obesity – pathophysiological concepts and effects of physical activity. Dtsch Z Sportmed. 2017;68:163-69.

24. Kawanishi N, Yano H, Yokogawa Y, Suzuki K. Exercise training inhibits inflammation in adipose tissue via both suppression of macrophage infiltration and acceleration of phenotypic switching from M1 to M2 macrophages in high-fat-diet-induced obese mice. Exerc Immunol Rev. 2010;16:105-18.

Chapter 11
Vitamin D and musculoskeletal health

As you read in the previous chapter, as our body fat mass becomes obese, fat cells begin to function in a pro-inflammatory fashion and anti-inflammatory immune cells are replaced by pro-inflammatory immune cells. This can lead many to believe that their immune systems are anti-inflammatory if they are not overweight or obese, which is not necessarily true.

It is certainly possible for me to eat 60% of my calories from refined sugar, flour, and omega-6 oils, and still keep my overall caloric intake at a level that does not cause me to gain weight. If I did this, I would still be deficient in potassium, magnesium, iodine, omega-3 fatty acids, polyphenols, carotenoids, and assuming I avoided sun exposure, I would also be deficient in vitamin D. If I were to do this, then my immune system would behave in a pro-inflammatory fashion that is similar to that which occurs in obese adipose tissue, a topic that was discussed in the previous chapter.

Vitamin D deficiency and related supplementation has become extremely popular in the last 15-20 years. Research has identified that multiple diseases are promoted by a chronic deficiency of vitamin D. Table 1 below is from *The DeFlame Diet* book, which highlights many of the conditions related to a deficiency of vitamin D. Notice that the first nine conditions in the left column demonstrate the importance of vitamin D for musculoskeletal function.

Table 1 - Potential consequences of vitamin D deficiency

Muscle aches	Influenza
Muscle weakness	Schizophrenia
Osteoarthritis	Depression
Osteoporosis	Metabolic syndrome
Rickets	Type 2 diabetes
Osteomalacia (bone pain)	Tuberculosis
Back pain	Common cold
Pseudofractures	Bacterial vaginosis
Widespread pain	Ulcerative colitis
Asthma	Rheumatoid arthritis
Cardiovascular disease	Parkinson's disease
Hypertension	Alzheimer's
Epilepsy	Breast cancer
Type 1 diabetes	Prostate cancer
Multiple sclerosis	Colon cancer
Crohn's disease	Pancreatic cancer

Like obesity, a lack of vitamin D increases inflammation by increasing the number of pro-inflammatory immune cells in circulation that release the various pro-inflammatory cytokines. So, if a person is obese and vitamin D deficient, which is quite common, then the vitamin D deficiency state will augment the pro-inflammatory state of obesity. If one is not obese, but is deficient in vitamin D, this will lead to an increased number of pro-inflammatory immune cells and a reduction of anti-inflammatory immune cells in body circulation.

Figure 1 in this chapter illustrates the same pro- and anti-inflammatory T-lymphocytes that were discussed in the previous chapter about obesity. Th0 cells are T-helper precursor cells, which differentiate into T-helper 1 cells (Th1), T-helper 2 cells (Th2), T-helper 17 cells (Th17), and T-regulatory cells (Treg).

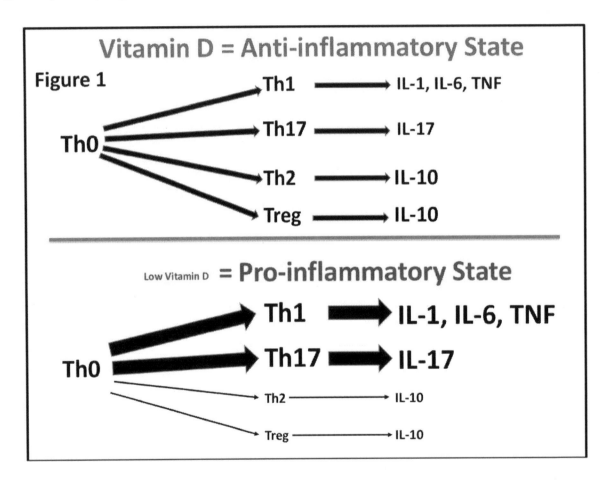

Th1 and Th17 cells promote inflammation by releasing pro-inflammatory cytokines, such as interleukin-1 (IL-1), interleukin-6 (IL-6), interleukin-17 (IL-17), and tumor necrosis factor (TNF). Th2 and Treg cells inhibit inflammation by releasing interleukin-10 (IL-10), the key anti-inflammatory cytokine. For a normal, healthy DeFlamed state of immunity, we need a proper balance between the pro-inflammatory and anti-inflammatory cells and their respective cytokines. Pro-inflammatory cytokines are involved in the injury response, whether it be a traumatic event or an infection. The pro-inflammatory cytokine response should be short-lived and then replaced by the anti-inflammatory cytokine healing response.

When there is an imbalance in cytokine production, it is never shifted toward being too anti-inflammatory, which means the balance problem always shifts toward being pro-inflammatory. This means that we should not engage in behaviors that inhibit our anti-inflammatory T-cells to shift us into a pro-inflammatory state.

From a practical perspective, we can view any unhealthy lifestyle choice as a promoter of pro-inflammatory immune responses and an inhibitor of anti-inflammatory immune responses. This is obviously a very general statement and not so easy to visualize. Fortunately, vitamin D and immune cell function has been studied by scientists so we can create a visual image to never forget how this works. Figure 1 illustrates what happens to immune cell expression when there is adequate and inadequate levels of vitamin D (1-3).

Notice in Figure 1 that Th0 cells are the precursors to all the other T-cells. Th0 cells are referred to as naïve cells, which have the capacity to become both anti-inflammatory Th2 and Treg cells or pro-inflammatory Th1 and Th17 cells. Notice that when there is adequate vitamin D, we get a balanced production of T-cells. However, when we are deficient in vitamin D, Th0 cells are converted into pro-inflammatory T-cells.

Recall from the end of Chapter 10 of this book that the pro-inflammatory cytokines (IL-1, IL-6, IL-17, and TNF) that are overproduced in obesity, participate in the rotting degradation of muscles, joints, tendons, spinal discs and bones. The same cytokines are overproduced during vitamin D deficiency, which promotes the same degradative outcome. This is how obesity and vitamin D deficiency deliver a double degradative hit to our musculoskeletal tissues.

If that was not bad enough, we also know that an inadequate intake of magnesium and omega-3 fatty acids creates a similar pro-inflammatory immune cell profile as obesity and vitamin D deficiency (4,5). In other words, we suffer cumulative pro-inflammatory "hits" when we adopt an unhealthy lifestyle, all of which lead to a degeneration and rotting of musculoskeletal tissues, which causes pain, weakness, and movement restrictions.

This is why the DeFlame approach to diet is about addressing and monitoring the inflammatory markers listed in Chapter 3 of this book. If we normalize all of the inflammatory markers, we have a much better chance of protecting and preserving the function of our musculoskeletal tissues. In the context of this chapter, most experts agree that we should get our vitamin D level tested, as measured by 25(OH)D in a blood test. The goal, as described in *The DeFlame Diet* book, should be to reach 70 ng/ml.

References

1. Cantorna MT, Mahon BD. Mounting evidence for vitamin D as an environmental factor affecting autoimmune disease prevalence. Exp Biol Med. 2004; 229:1136-42.
2. Cantorna MT, Snyder L, Lin YD, Yang L. Vitamin D and 1,25(OH)2D regulation of T cells. Nutrients. 2015;7:3011-21.

3. Arnson Y, Amital H, Shoenfeld Y. Vitamin D and autoimmunity: a new aetiological and therapeutic considerations. Ann Rheum Dis. 2007;66:1137-42.

4. Chung HS, Park CS, Hong SH, et al. Effects of magnesium pretreatment on the levels of T helper cytokines and on the severity of reperfusion syndrome in patients undergoing living donor liver transplantation. Magnesium Res. 2013;26:46-55.

5. Hichami A, Grissa O, Mrizak I, et al. Role of T-cell polarization and inflammation and their modulation by n-3 fatty acids in gestational diabetes and macrosomia. J Nutr Metab. 2016; Article ID:3124960.

Chapter 12
Metabolic syndrome: A state of systemic body rot

In Chapter 3, I indicated that the metabolic syndrome is a driver of chronic pain and the degeneration of muscles, tendons, joints, spinal discs, and bones. In other words, the metabolic syndrome causes our body to rot. This chapter represents a deeper dive into the nature of the metabolic syndrome so that you can better understand how it promotes a rotting state in our musculoskeletal tissues.

As stated in Chapter 3, in order to be diagnosed with the metabolic syndrome, you need at least 3 of the 5 markers in Table 1 with an abnormal value. Approximately 25% of all adults in the United States have the metabolic syndrome. This number rises to about 45% of adults over the age of 60 (1,2).

Table 1 - Metabolic syndrome markers

Metabolic syndrome	Abnormal value	Date	Date	Date	Date
1. Fasting blood glucose	≥ 100 mg/dL				
2. Fasting triglycerides	≥ 150 mg/dL				
3. Fasting HDL cholesterol	< 50 for women; < 40 men				
4. Blood pressure	≥ 130/85				
5. Waist circumference	> 35″ women; > 40″ men				

The hallmark sign of the metabolic syndrome and diabetes is elevated blood glucose levels. The reason why glucose levels rise is because skeletal muscles are no longer able to properly take up circulating glucose. Chronic inflammation causes skeletal muscles to become insulin resistant, which is why the metabolic syndrome is also called the insulin resistance syndrome. Both the metabolic syndrome and type 2 diabetes are insulin resistant conditions, it is just way worse with type 2 diabetes. Another feature of insulin resistance is increased blood levels of insulin, called hyperinsulinemia. The next several paragraphs describe how skeletal muscle become insulin resistant.

Normally, when blood glucose levels rise, the pancreas releases an appropriate amount of insulin, which binds to its receptor on the membrane of skeletal muscle and leads to the uptake of glucose. There are several steps between the binding of insulin to its receptor on skeletal muscle and the subsequent uptake of glucose. Once insulin binds, it is supposed to trigger a domino effect or chain reaction, which involves several steps that occur within skeletal muscle, which ultimately leads to muscle uptake of glucose. Understand that it is skeletal muscle that is the primary organ/tissue that takes in glucose after a meal. In fact, 80% of glucose uptake is done by skeletal muscle (3). This process works well until people begin to overeat refined sugar, flour, and oil calories, become obese and insulin resistant.

Initially, when we are young, overeating refined carbohydrates will stimulate the pancreas to release excess insulin. Assuming an individual is healthy, this process allows for blood glucose to remain at a normal level because skeletal muscle rapidly takes up the excess glucose. But over time, this changes due to the development of obesity.

The chronic systemic inflammation created by fat cells and immune cells in obese adipose tissue inhibits the insulin signaling chain reaction in skeletal muscles and prevents them from taking up glucose. In other words, the inflammatory cytokines released by obese adipose tissue cells enters body circulation and causes skeletal muscle to become resistant to the stimulatory effects of insulin, which is referred to as insulin resistance. At this stage, the ongoing pattern of overeating sugar, flour, oils, and fat continues to create hyperglycemia, hyperlipemia, and hyperinsulinemia; however, due the insulin resistance in skeletal muscle, the hyperglycemia and hyperinsulinemia gets worse.

The outcome of skeletal muscle insulin resistance is higher levels of blood glucose (hyperglycemia), which leads to more insulin release by the pancreas. Despite increased blood levels of insulin, skeletal muscles nonetheless remain resistant to insulin's actions because of the ongoing systemic chronic inflammatory state created by obese adipose tissue. Additionally, skeletal muscles begin to store an excess of triglycerides and additional pro-inflammatory fats, which also causes muscles to become insulin resistant. The outcome is ever-rising levels of blood glucose, which causes body cells to overproduce and release pro-inflammatory chemicals into body circulation as described in Chapter 6, which serves to rot our musculoskeletal tissues.

At this point in the book, it should be clear that hyperglycemia is pro-inflammatory because it induces cells in the body to pump out pro-inflammatory chemicals. Hyperglycemia has an additional pro-inflammatory effect that you should know about. Because glucose levels are perpetually elevated in the metabolic syndrome and diabetes, this leads to a type of tissue sugar-coating, which is called glycation. The most well-known example of this is glycated hemoglobin, called hemoglobin A1c. Anyone with the metabolic syndrome or diabetes typically knows their A1c level, which should be below 5.7%. Hemoglobin is a protein and excess glucose in circulation binds to hemoglobin. Excess glucose also binds to lipids, such as LDL cholesterol. The term advanced glycation end products (AGEs) refers to any protein or lipid that has been glycated. An excess of AGEs is known to promote chronic inflammation and body rot. AGEs will be discussed more in upcoming chapters.

If you look at Table 1 at the beginning of the chapter, you will notice that hyperinsulinemia is not one of the criteria for the metabolic syndrome. A reason is because when someone has hyperglycemia, hypertriglyceridemia, and low HDL cholesterol, we know that this individual will also have hyperinsulinemia. The primary difference between the metabolic syndrome and type 2 diabetes is the level of fasting glucose and postprandial (post-eating) glucose. As stated earlier in this chapter, both conditions are associated with insulin resistance in skeletal muscle and hyperinsulinemia…it is just way worse with type 2 diabetes, which also means type 2 diabetics have higher levels of glucose and triglycerides, and lower levels of HDL cholesterol.

The pro-inflammatory effects of hyperglycemia have been discussed in previous chapters and in great detail in *The DeFlame Diet* book. You should also know about the pro-inflammatory effects of hyperinsulinemia.

Insulin is typically viewed as the hormone that regulates blood glucose levels, which is true; however, there are additional important pro-inflammatory functions that you should know about as insulin levels rise above normal. Hyperinsulinemia stimulates fat production by a process called lipogenesis, which means fat creation from glucose which we get from overeating refined sugar and flour. This occurs largely in fat cells and the liver. The outcome is an excess of fat storage in fat cells and the liver, and also causes fat levels in the blood to rise and leads to increased fat storage in other tissues, most notably in skeletal muscle, which is part of the rotting process that occurs in skeletal muscle.

One of the fats that is produced by the liver and fat cells from glucose is a saturated fatty acid called palmitate or palmitic acid. Not surprisingly, this means that excess palmitate circulates in the blood stream of people who are insulin resistant. Palmitate is taken up by skeletal muscles and converted into a pro-inflammatory fat called ceramide, a process that correlates directly to hyperinsulinemia and insulin resistance (4,5). Ceramide and its muscle rotting effects will be discussed more in Chapter 14.

Hyperinsulinemia is also directly related to problems related to cholesterol synthesis. Since at least the 1980s (6), and perhaps earlier, it has been known that hyperinsulinemia causes an overproduction of LDL cholesterol and an underproduction of HDL cholesterol, and the subsequent free radicalization of both LDL and HDL cholesterol. This topic will be discussed more in Chapter 13.

In short, when you see the term "insulin resistance," that should make you think hyperglycemia, hyperlipemia, and hyperinsulinemia, which represents a robust pro-inflammatory state and correlates with the development of obesity and overall body rot.

In the context of this current chapter, you should also know that a deficiency of vitamin D is a considered a promoter of insulin resistance (7-9), which is another reason why we should all get our vitamin D levels to an optimal level.

C-reactive protein (CRP) was also discussed in Chapter 3. As metabolic syndrome markers rise into the abnormal range, so do CRP levels, which means that insulin resistance correlates to CRP levels (10). It is not uncommon for physicians to measure CRP levels, which is typically done in the context of concerns about cardiovascular disease. While CRP levels are certainly predictive of cardiovascular health, you should understand that CRP is not specific to cardiovascular health…CRP is an inflammatory protein and reflects overall body inflammation, which is the key promoter for all chronic diseases and is associated with the degeneration of musculoskeletal tissues.

A normal CRP level is below 1.0 mg/L, which should be the goal for all of us. An individual is considered to be moderately inflamed, or rotting, if their CRP level is between 1-3 mg/L. The average adult American has a CRP level of 1.5 mg/L, which means the average adult in America spends 24 hours per day in the moderately rotting category. If CRP levels rise above 3 mg/L, the individual is considered to be highly inflamed or rotting. It turns out that about 25% of adult Americans have CRP levels above 3 mg/L (11), which means that a full 25% of Americans aged 20 and older are literally rotting from chronic inflammation.

The pro-inflammatory metabolic syndrome can also be viewed as a "free radical" state, wherein the production of free radicals outpaces their reduction by the body's built in antioxidant system, which was described in Chapter 8. Antioxidant supplements are also unable to adequately counteract the free radical state of the metabolic syndrome.

The state of immune activity in people with the metabolic syndrome has also been studied. Due to the presence of such pro-inflammatory factors as obesity, hyperglycemia, AGEs, and oxidized LDL, the metabolic syndrome is characterized as a state of "maladaptive chronic non-resolving immune activation" (12), which in common language means "a rotting body."

As almost 60% of the average American's diet consists of refined sugar, flour, and omega-6 oil calories, it should not be a surprise that this is the eating problem that causes the metabolic syndrome to emerge. The DeFlame Diet approach is to avoid these calories to achieve normal markers of inflammation, which means you can do it as a vegan, omnivore, or carnivore. I favor the omnivore diet (meat, fish, chicken, and vegetation). Whichever you prefer, let the normalization and maintenance of the inflammation markers be your dietary guide, rather than an alleged authority who claims you can only eat a certain way.

In subsequent chapters, you will see how the metabolic syndrome, which means hyperglycemia, hyperlipemia, hyperinsulinemia, and insulin resistance, creates a pro-inflammatory state that promotes a rotting process in muscles, joints, tendons, spinal discs, and bones. Regarding joints specifically, scientists have proposed that osteoarthritis be considered a component of the metabolic syndrome (13). Before discussing the various musculoskeletal tissues, we need to consider cardiovascular disease, because without cardiovascular health, it is very difficult to engage in physical activities.

References

1. Ford ES, Giles WH, Dietz WH. Prevalence of the metabolic syndrome among US adults. Findings from the Third National Health and Nutrition Examination Survey. J Am Med Assoc. 200; 287:356-59.

2. Ford ES. Prevalence of the metabolic syndrome defined by the International Diabetes Federation among adults in the U.S. Diabetes Care. 2005;28(11):2745-49.

3. Tumova J, Andel M, Trnka J. Excess free fatty acids as a cause of metabolic dysfunction in skeletal muscle. Physiol Res. 2016;65:193-207.

4. Hansen ME, Tippetts TS, Anderson MC. Insulin increases ceramide synthesis in skeletal muscle. J Diabetes Res. 2014; Article ID: 765784.

5. Turpin SM, Lancaster GI, Darby I, Febbraio MA, Watt MJ. Apoptosis in skeletal myotubes is induced by ceramides and is positively related to insulin resistance. Am J Physiol Endocrinol Metab. 2006;291:E1341-50.

6. Fossati P, Romon-Rousseax M. Insulin and HDL-cholesterol metabolism. Diabete Metab. 1987;13(3 Pt 2):390-94.

7. Schwalfenberg G. Vitamin D and diabetes: improvement of glycemic control with vitamin D3 repletion. Can Fam Phys. 2008;54:864-66.

8. Mezza T, Muscogiuri G, Sorice GP, et al. Vitamin D deficiency: a new risk factor for type 2 diabetes? Ann Nutr Metab. 2012;61:337-48.

9. Curmaz AH, Demir AD, Ozkan T. Does vitamin D deficiency lead to insulin resistance in obese individuals. Biomed Res. 2017;28:7491-97.

10. Yudkin JS, Stehouwer CD, Emeis JJ, Coppack SW. C-reactive protein in healthy subjects: associations with obesity, insulin resistance, and endothelial dysfunction. A potential role for cytokines originating form adipose tissue? Arterioscler Thromb Vasc Biol. 1999;19:972-78.

11. Ridker PM. Cardiology patient page. C-reactive protein: a simple test to help predict risk of heart attack and stroke. Circulation 2003, 108:81–85.

12. Zmora N, Bashiades S, Levy M, Elinav E. The role of the immune system in metabolic health and disease. 2017;25:508-21.

13. Zhuo Q, Yang W, Chen J, Wang Y. Metabolic syndrome meets osteoarthritis. Nat Rev Rheumatol. 2012;8:729-37.

68

Chapter 13
Atherosclerosis: Diet-induced vascular rot

Without adequate cardiovascular health it can be a challenge to engage in physical activities. This has become especially obvious to me at the golf course or at the beach, where flamed up people are huffing and puffing while they walk around or try to negotiate mild waves. It is so bad that many people can barely walk through Sam's Club or IKEA without feeling like they are going to have a heart attack.

From a pathology perspective, it turns out that the diet-induced inflammation and degeneration, i.e., the rotting process, that take place in blood vessels with atherosclerosis is essentially identical to the rotting process that takes place in musculoskeletal tissues. So, understanding the pro-inflammatory atherosclerotic rotting process will help you to understand the pro-inflammatory processes that occur in musculoskeletal tissues. Oftentimes, both processes progress together, which is important to know. It is also important to know that a DeFlamed diet and lifestyle will prevent each from developing and can help to reverse the process by eliminating the dietary drive that serves as a key promotional factor.

The following terms are used when referring to the narrowing or blockage of blood arteries in the heart: atherosclerosis, atherosclerotic vascular disease, cardiovascular disease, heart disease, and angina. Vascular disease refers to disease of the arteries or veins, but it is most commonly used in everyday language when referring to atherosclerosis in arteries. The most important point to understand about atherosclerosis is that it is a chronic pro-inflammatory state within the walls of arteries (1,2), which should be viewed as a rotting process. The same atherosclerotic rotting process occurs in heart arteries, which can cause a heart attack, in brain arteries, which can cause a stroke, and in peripheral arteries (in the pelvic/thigh region), which is called peripheral artery disease (PAD) that causes leg pain while walking.

As indicated in the previous paragraph, atherosclerosis only occurs in certain arteries; not in other arteries and NEVER in veins. This fact should actually make us question the validity of the notion that eating saturated fat and cholesterol is the cause of atherosclerosis. Consider that when you go for a blood test, from which vessel is blood drawn? The answer is a vein, NOT an artery. This is important to understand because your cholesterol level is the same in both veins and arteries, yet it is ONLY arteries that suffer from atherosclerosis.

With the above information in mind, why do you think it is that we only get atherosclerosis in arteries and NOT in veins? The answer is because the curves and bifurcations of only certain arteries, such as coronary arteries, brain arteries, and pelvic/thigh arteries, causes them to be constantly exposed to pro-inflammatory turbulent forces created by the pumping of blood by the heart. In contrast, veins throughout the body are NEVER exposed to these turbulent forces and so veins NEVER develop atherosclerosis, with one exception. The scenario wherein veins do develop atherosclerosis is when a vein is used to replace a diseased coronary artery. Within a short period of time, the transplanted vein will develop atherosclerosis due to the fact that this vein must now deal with pro-inflammatory turbulent forces that it NEVER dealt with when it was part of the venous system (3). It should be clear that the pro-inflammatory turbulence in arteries is the cause of atherosclerosis and NOT cholesterol levels.

It turns out that arteries have a built-in anti-inflammatory mechanism for dealing with pro-inflammatory turbulence to prevent the development of atherosclerosis; however, this capacity is lost in people who live on a pro-inflammatory diet. To appreciate how this works, some basic artery anatomy and physiology should be understood.

Look at Figure 1, which illustrates the differences between arteries and veins. Very small arteries are called arterioles and very small veins are called venules. The artery system brings oxygen-rich blood to musculoskeletal and visceral organs and the venous system returns that blood to the lungs to get more oxygen. Capillaries are the smallest of our vessels. They serve as the interface between arteries and veins, and are also responsible for delivering oxygen-rich blood and nutrients to our tissues.

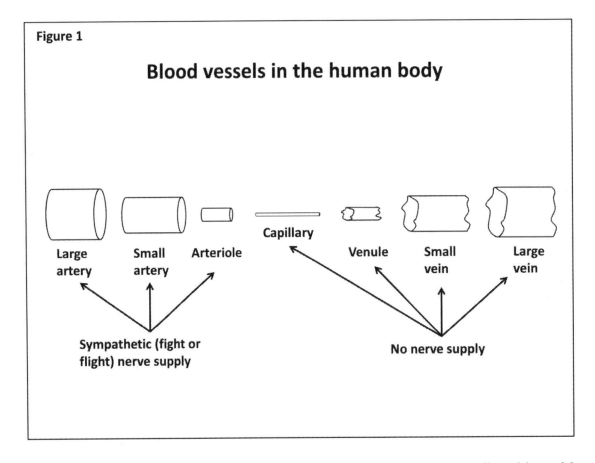

Figure 1

Blood vessels in the human body

Notice that veins look different than arteries. In the body, veins are more collapsible and have a flattened appearance compared to arteries which appear round. This is because arteries have thicker walls compared to the thin walls of veins, which allows for arteries to withstand greater pressures and pro-inflammatory turbulent forces compared to veins.

Notice also in Figure 1 that there is no nerve supply to capillaries and veins. In contrast, arteries do have a nerve supply that causes arteries to constrict. A blood pressure of less than 120/80 reflects normal tone within the artery system. When blood pressure rises above normal, arteries are forced to deal with greater pressure and more pro-inflammatory turbulence, which is why high blood pressure promotes atherosclerosis.

Figure 2 illustrates the various layers in the wall of an artery and arteriole. Tunica means a layer. Arteries and veins both have three layers; however, arteries have a much larger muscular layer. The inner layer is called the tunica intima, which contains endothelial cells. Below the endothelial cell layer is a layer of connective tissue and below that is the internal elastic membrane, which are components of the tunica intimate that give it support and structure, but are not illustrated in Figure 2. The middle layer is called the tunica media, which contains the smooth muscle cells, which can contract or relax to increase and decrease artery pressure. The outer layer is called the tunica adventitia or externa, which contains connective tissue that is made of collagen, much like that which you find in muscles, joints, tendons, spinal discs, and in skin for the purpose of providing these tissues with structure.

Figure 2

Artery anatomy

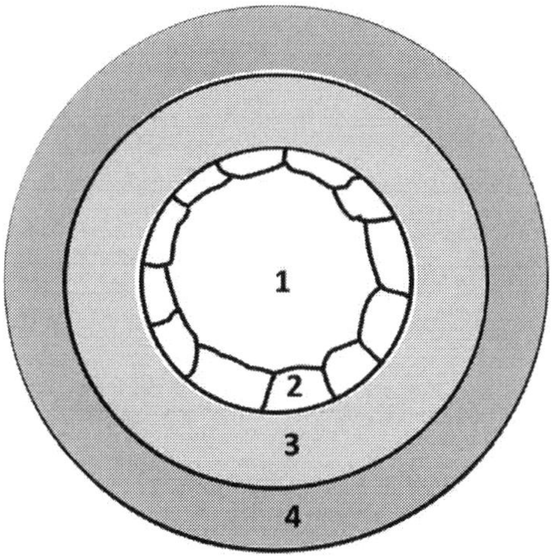

1. **Lumen**
2. **Tunica intima (endothelial cell layer)**
3. **Tunica media (smooth muscle cell layer)**
4. **Tunica adventitia or externa (connective tissue layer)**

Until the last couple of decades, endothelial cells were viewed as merely the inner lining of arteries and arterioles, and that they served no biological function. We now know that this view was quite oversimplified.

It turns out that part of the job of the endothelial cell is to direct the activity of the smooth muscle cells in artery walls. Here is how it works. Endothelial cells normally produce a substance called nitric oxide, which causes smooth muscle cells to have an anti-inflammatory relaxation response to pro-inflammatory turbulence and pressure. Before it was identified to be nitric oxide, scientists referred to it as endothelial-derived relaxing factor. An enzyme called endothelial nitric oxide synthase (eNOS) is responsible for producing nitric oxide, which then causes artery smooth muscle to DeFlame and relax. Not surprisingly, free radicals and pro-inflammatory cytokines inhibit eNOS, which impairs artery relaxation and promotes both atherosclerosis and high blood pressure (4,5).

While free radicals impair eNOS, the anti-inflammatory dietary polyphenols (pigments in vegetables and fruit) support the production of eNOS (6). Scientists have referred to these anti-inflammatory polyphenols as vasodilating or vasorelaxing polyphenols (7,8), which means they participate in the anti-inflammatory response to pro-inflammatory turbulence, which prevents atherosclerosis from developing.

Dietary potassium also helps arteries to relax. A lack of potassium in endothelial cells impairs artery relaxation, promotes local inflammation, promotes free radical generation, and promotes atherosclerosis and high blood pressure (9-12).

Omega-3 fatty acids have long been known to help relax arteries and to reduce inflammation in the artery walls (13,14). In addition to nitric oxide, endothelial cells produce another vasorelaxing substance called prostacyclin that comes from dietary omega-6 and omega-3 fatty acids.

All cells, including endothelial cells and smooth muscle cells can produce pro-inflammatory chemicals in excess when the diet and other lifestyle choices are pro-inflammatory. In the case of endothelial cells, it has been known for many years that they will release an excess of pro-inflammatory chemicals (free radicals, cytokines, growth factors, adhesion molecules, and a prostaglandin-like substance made from omega-6 fatty acids called thromboxane A2) that function to promote atherosclerosis (15).

A pro-inflammatory diet also causes an immune cell population shift to occur in artery walls. A normal artery has anti-inflammatory immune cells, which help to prevent atherosclerosis (16). However, a pro-inflammatory diet causes pro-inflammatory immune cells to accumulate within vessel walls to begin producing pro-inflammatory chemicals and they recruit additional pro-inflammatory immune cells to enter the vessel wall to perpetuate the atherosclerotic rotting process (2,16). The pro-inflammatory immune cell profile in atherosclerotic arteries is the same as that in obese adipose tissue as illustrated in Chapter 10. Figure 3 in this chapter illustrates the accumulation of pro-inflammatory immune cells within the vessel wall, including pro-inflammatory M1 macrophages, T-helper 1 (Th1) cells, and T-helper 17 (Th17) cells. Foam cells are macrophages that have engulfed oxidized LDL cholesterol, which will be discussed more below.

Figure 3 also includes the various pro-inflammatory factors that impact artery walls to promote atherosclerosis, most of which have been discussed previously in this book including, hyperglycemia, free radicals (FR), advanced glycation end products (AGEs), omega-6 fatty acids (n-6), endotoxin, and cytokines. Notice that the vascular wall is also compromised by MMPs and oxLDL, which will be discussed next.

MMPs is the acronym for a family of connective tissue digesting enzymes called matrix metalloproteinases. When the dietary flame goes on, these enzymes can no longer be properly regulated, causing too much collagen degradation in artery walls, which adds to the atherosclerotic rotting process. MMPs will be discussed in more detail in Chapters 15-17, as they also participate in osteoarthritis, tendinosis, and disc herniation.

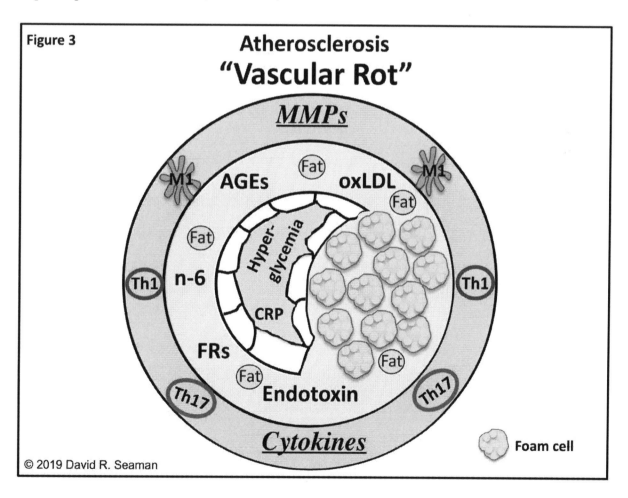

Figure 3

Atherosclerosis "Vascular Rot"

© 2019 David R. Seaman

The final pro-inflammatory chemical to be discussed in Figure 3 is oxLDL, which means oxidized, or free radicalized, LDL cholesterol. There is a reason why I have not mentioned cholesterol up to this point in this chapter. People need to understand that it is possible to discuss atherosclerosis without focusing on cholesterol. In fact, cholesterol does not cause heart disease in the simplistic and sophomoric fashion that has been presented to us over the many decades (3). For more details about how this works, check out *The DeFlame Diet* book that contains about 45 pages devoted to fats, triglycerides, and cholesterol. What follows is an abbreviated version of the cholesterol story that I wrote about in *The DeFlame Diet*.

Consider that in the normal state, the liver produces more LDL cholesterol than HDL cholesterol; just look at the ranges for LDL and HDL on your most recent blood test. If it were true that LDL cholesterol is so bad, why would the liver normally produce more of it than the so-called good HDL cholesterol? In short, it is a preposterous notion to suggest that LDL cholesterol is bad. It turns out that both LDL and HDL cholesterol are normally anti-inflammatory; however, they become pro-inflammatory and disease promoting when one adopts a high calorie, pro-inflammatory diet. Figure 4 illustrates this process.

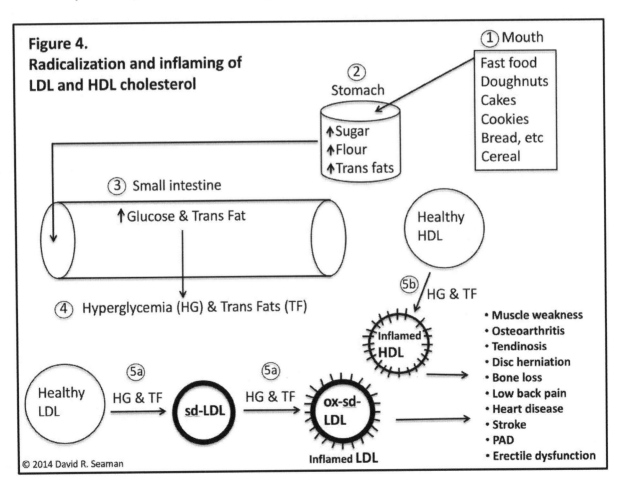

When we are young and healthy, our LDL and HDL cholesterol are both healthy and DeFlamed. In this state, LDL does not cause heart disease or any other problem; however, this changes over time wherein both LDL and HDL become inflamed and cause disease. Figure 4 on the last page illustrates this process. As stated previously in this book, the average American gets almost 60% of their calories from refined sugar, flour, and omega-6 oils. We also consume trans fats, which should never be consumed. We get these refined calories from the "foods" listed in box #1. In the stomach, these foods are broken down into their constituent parts, those being sugar, flour, and trans fats, which are then sent into the small intestine.

The sugar and flour become glucose and then the glucose along with the trans fats are absorbed into the blood stream. Doing this once in while is no big deal; however, about 70% of Americans are overweight or obese, which means most people overeat these refined calories on a regular basis. Over time, this leads to the development of the metabolic syndrome. Recall from Chapter 3 and 12, which also listed the markers of the metabolic syndrome in Table 1.

Table 1 - Metabolic syndrome markers

Metabolic syndrome	Abnormal value	Date	Date	Date	Date
1. Fasting blood glucose	≥ 100 mg/dL				
2. Fasting triglycerides	≥ 150 mg/dL				
3. Fasting HDL cholesterol	< 50 for women; < 40 men				
4. Blood pressure	≥ 130/85				
5. Waist circumference	> 35" women; > 40" men				

The pro-inflammatory metabolic syndrome causes HDL and LDL to become pro-inflammatory. HDL is also transformed into an inflamed state by chronic hyperglycemia and trans fats. Normally, the healthy DeFlamed version of HDL helps to keep LDL in a DeFlamed state, but this function is lost due to chronic hyperglycemia and trans fats.

In the case of LDL, it is normally large and buoyant, which means that it is DeFlamed. Chronic hyperglycemia (HG) and trans fats (TF) first mutate the large buoyant LDL into one that is small and dense (sd-LDL), but it does not stop there. The sd-LDL is then oxidized (ox-sd-LDL) and so it is referred to as oxidized LDL, which is recognized by the immune system as a pathogen. Part of the bodily process for eliminating pathogens is for macrophages to engulf and remove them from circulation. Foam cells are macrophages that have engulfed pathogenic oxidized LDL. Foam cells accumulate in an unrelenting fashion in rotting atherosclerotic vessels so long as oxidized LDL continues to be produced and requires removal. Thus, the so-called "build-up" of cholesterol in atherosclerotic vessels is actually represented by the accumulation of foam cells as illustrated in Figure 3.

So, it is NOT regular LDL that is problematic. Regular LDL has no disease-promoting potential when it is soft and buoyant. For LDL to cause heart disease, it must be transformed into one that is small, dense, and oxidized. It is this inflamed version of LDL that causes atherosclerosis and subsequently heart disease, strokes, PAD, and even erectile dysfunction (17,18).

Not well known is the fact that oxidized LDL cholesterol also promotes musculoskeletal conditions, including muscle weakness (19,20), osteoarthritis (21), tendinopathy (22), disc herniation and low back pain (23,24), and bone loss (25,26). The next several chapters will look at individual musculoskeletal tissues and outline how a pro-inflammatory diet causes them to degenerate and become painful.

How do you know if your LDL cholesterol is oxidized? The challenge is that testing for oxidized LDL is done in the research setting and not in the patient care setting, so here is how we can determine if LDL is oxidized without actually testing for it directly. If you have the metabolic syndrome (see Table 1), this means you have the pro-inflammatory state that promotes the oxidation of LDL. More specifically, an indirect measurement of oxidized LDL can be determined by dividing your fasting triglyceride level by your fasting HDL cholesterol level, which gives you the ratio of fasting triglycerides to HDL. If this ratio is greater than 3.5, it is essentially guaranteed that your oxidized LDL level is abnormally high and capable of causing all the problems listed in Figure 4. Ideally the triglyceride/HDL ratio should be less than 2, which can be achieved by DeFlaming the diet and becoming physically active.

If you are taking a statin for your cholesterol level, the clinical decision was not based on a measurement of your oxidized LDL level; it was most likely based on your regular LDL level and your total cholesterol level. What you likely were not told is that insulin levels rise when we overeat sugar and flour and become overweight and obese, and it is insulin that stimulates the key enzyme in cholesterol production, called HMG-CoA reductase. This is the same enzyme that statins inhibit, which is described in more detail in *The DeFlame Diet* book. For our purposes here, you should understand that most people can be weaned off of statins, so long as they DeFlame their diets and get all of their markers back to normal.

The problem with long-term use of statins is that they can have many side effects that are not beneficial for people who wish to be physically active, the most notable and well known is muscle pain. For many years we have known about additional problematic symptoms that can emerge with long term statin use, such as fatigue, memory loss, cognitive defects, irritability and aggression, and neuropathies (27-30). My suggestion is to get DeFlamed so your medical doctor does not feel the need to prescribe you a statin or can wean you off of it, so you can avoid these potential side effects that can compromise your musculoskeletal system and prevent you from engaging in the activities you love.

Lipid accumulation in atherosclerosis

While lipids (fats) do accumulate in an atherosclerotic artery, it is more complicated than the simplistic view we have told. The traditional story that doctors were taught was that fat and cholesterol build up on the endothelial layer, which eventually occludes the lumen so blood cannot flow properly, which causes a heart attack, stroke, or peripheral artery disease. For many years, scientists have explained that lipids do not accumulate in this fashion (1,2,3), but this has yet to permeate in the clinical and public domains. Atherosclerosis is now known to be an inflammatory state within the vessel wall (1,3), which is also where lipids are found.

Unlike what you might think, lipid does not accumulate as layers of saturated fat and cholesterol. The lipid content of an atherosclerotic artery correlates to the presence of activated macrophages (31). These macrophages engulf oxidized LDL cholesterol because it is perceived to be similar to any other pathogen. As stated earlier in this chapter, the term foam cell is used to describe these lipid-filled macrophages that accumulate within the vessel wall. While there are lipids in the vessel wall, the vast majority of lipids found in the vessel wall are actually inside macrophages.

Saturated fatty acids also participate in atherosclerosis, but like cholesterol, it does not work the way you would think based on the propaganda we have been fed about this topic. In the previous chapter, I described how excess glucose from overeating refined sugar and flour gets converted into an excessive amount of a saturated fatty acid called palmitic acid. Excess palmitic acid enters the vessel wall and stimulates smooth muscle cells to release inflammatory cytokines and other chemicals that promote atherosclerosis (32). Clearly, the true saturated fat problem has little to do with eating foods with saturated fatty acids.

In subsequent chapters, you will see how oxidized LDL cholesterol and palmitic acid participate in promoting musculoskeletal conditions. In short, lipids accumulate in muscles, joints, and tendons, which demonstrates that musculoskeletal conditions are biologically very similar to atherosclerosis.

How a heart attack is like joint and tendon pain

This section describes a concept that is very important to understand. Practitioners in the medical, physical therapy, and chiropractic world tend to view osteoarthritis and tendon pathology (called tendinopathy or tendinosis) as "wear and tear" conditions. The proper view is that they are "wear and lack of repair" conditions, which will be explained in more detail in the upcoming joint and tendon chapters.

For now, consider a 45-year old man who is 50 pounds overweight. He decides to eat better and exercise to get his weight back to normal. He goes out for a run and has a heart attack. No one would jump to the conclusion that exercise is the cause of heart disease or a heart attack. Everyone would properly conceptualize that the guy was too overweight to run and likely had atherosclerotic heart disease, which was not symptomatic at rest. When he ran, the rotted (inflamed) and narrowed arteries were unable to deliver blood and oxygen to the heart, so he had a heart attack. In other words, the cause of the heart attack was chronic inflammation of his coronary (heart) arteries; NOT exercise. This same perception should be applied to a different overweight 45-year old guy who developed joint or tendon pain after running.

We now know that joints and tendons undergo a chronic inflammatory rotting process that is almost identical to atherosclerosis (See Chapters 15 and 16). Just like atherosclerosis, osteoarthritis and tendinopathy develop without symptoms in people who are overweight, obese, and/or who have the metabolic syndrome. If our overweight, 45-year old guy decides to run on his symptom-free osteoarthritic joints or tendons with tendinopathy, this can bring out painful symptoms. This can lead a "wear and tear-thinking" clinician to misinterpret the emergence of the painful symptoms as being caused by the compressive and tensile loading created by running on otherwise normal joints and tendons. The proper interpretation is that the "pre-flamed" joints and tendons were simply unable to bear the normal load created by jogging. This issue will be described more in the respective chapters devoted to joints and tendons.

References

1. Libby P. Inflammation and cardiovascular disease mechanisms. Am J Clin Nutr. 2006;83(suppl):456S-60S.

2. Lamon BD, Hajjar DP. Inflammation at the molecular interface of atherogenesis. Am J Pathol. 2008;173:1253-64.

3. Stehbens WE. Hypothetical hypercholesterolemia and atherosclerosis. Med Hypoth. 2004;62:72-78.

4. Dinh QN, Drummond GR, Sobey CG, Chrissobolis S. Roles of inflammation, oxidative stress, and vascular dysfunction in hypertension. Biomed Res International. 2014; Article ID 406960.

5. Kawashima S, Yokoyama M. Dysfunction of endothelial nitric oxide synthase and atherosclerosis. Arterioscler Throm Vasc Biol. 2004;24:998-1005.

6. Nahas R. Complementary and alternative medicine approaches to blood pressure reduction: an evidence-based review. Can Fam Phys. 2008;54(11):1529-33.

7. Fitzpatrick DF Bing B, Maggi DA, Fleming RC, O'Malley RM. Vasodilating procyanidins derived from grape seeds. Ann NY Acad Sci. 2002;957:78-89.

8. Luna-Vasquez F, Ibarra-Alvarado C, Rojas-Molina A, Rojas-Molina I, Zavala-Sanchez MA. Vasodilator compounds derived from plants and their mechanisms of action. Molecules. 2013;18:5814-57.

9. Savage D, Perkins J, Hong Lim C, Bund SJ. Functional evidence that K+ is the non-nitric oxide, non-prostanoid endothelium-derived relaxing factor in rat femoral arteries. Vascul Pharmacol. 2003;40(1):23-28.

10. Kido M, Ando K, Onozato ML, et al. Protective effect of dietary potassium against vascular injury in salt-sensitive hypertension. Hypertension 2008;51;225-31.

11. Young DB, Ma G. Vascular protective effects of potassium. Semin Nephrol. 1999;19:477-86.

12. Young DB, Lin H, McCabe RD. Potassium's cardiovascular protective mechanisms. Am J Physiol. 1995;268(4 Pt 2):R825-37.

13. Simopoulos AP. Essential fatty acids in health and chronic disease. Am J Clin Nutr. 1999;70(suppl):560S-69S.

14. Holub BJ. Clinical nutrition: 4. Omega-3 fatty acids in cardiovascular care. Can Med Assoc J. 2002;166:608-15.

15. Cotran RS, Kumar V, Collins T. Robbins' Pathologic Basis of Disease. 6th ed. Philadelphia: WB Saunders; 1999: p.496.

16. Tabas I, Bornfeldt KE. Macrophage phenotype and function in different stages of atherosclerosis. Circ Res. 2016;118:653-67.

17. Vrentzos GE, Paraskevas KI, Mikhalidis DP. Dyslipidemia as a risk factor for erectile dysfunction. Curr Med Chem. 2007;14:1765-70.

18. Mitra S, Goyal T, Mehta JL. Oxidized LDL, LOX-1 and atherosclerosis. Cardiovascular Drugs Ther. 2011;25:419-29.

19. Kawamoto R, Kohara K, Katoh T, et al. Changes in oxidized low-density lipoprotein cholesterol are associated with changes in handgrip strength in Japanese community-dwelling persons. Endocrine. 2015;48:871-87.

20. Kawamoto R, Ninomiya D, Kasai Y, et al. Handgrip strength is associated with metabolic syndrome among middle-aged and elderly community-dwelling persons. Clin Exp Hypertens. 2016;38:245-51.

21. de Munter W, van der Kraon PM, van den Berg WB, van Lent PL. High systemic levels of low-density lipoprotein cholesterol: fuel to the flames of inflammatory osteoarthritis? Rheumatol. 2016;55:16-24.

22. Scott A, Zwerver J, Grewal N, et al. Lipids, adiposity and tendinopathy: is there a mechanistic link? Critical review. Br J Sports Med. 2015;49:984-88.

23. Li X, Wang X, Hu Z, et al. Possible involvement of the oxLDL/LOX-1 system in the pathogenesis and progression of human intervertebral disc degeneration or herniation. Scientific Reports. 2017;7:7403.

24. Kauppila LI. Atherosclerosis and disc degeneration/low back pain – a systematic review. Eur J Vasc Endovasc Surg. 2009;37:661-70.

25. Maziere C, Savitsky V, Galmiche A, et al. Oxidized low density lipoprotein inhibits phosphate signaling and phosphate-induced mineralization in osteoblasts. Involvement of oxidative stress. Biochim Biophys Acta. 2010;1802:1013-19.

26. Maziere C, Salle V, Gomila C, Maziere JC. Oxidized low density lipoprotein enhanced RANKL expression in human osteoblast-like cells. Involvement of ERK, NFkappaB and NFAT. Biochim Biophys Acta. 2013;1832:1756-64.

27. Golomb BA. Statin adverse effects: implications for the elderly. Geriatric Times. May/June 2004. http://www.geriatrictimes.com/g040618.html

28. Wagstaff LR, Mitton MW, Arvik BM, Doraiswamy PM. Statin-associated memory loss: analysis of 60 case reports and review of the literature. Pharmacotherapy 2003; 23(7):871-880.

29. Golomb BA, Kane T, Dimsdale JA (2004), Severe irritability associated with statin cholesterol-lowering drugs. QJM 97(4):229-235.

30. Gaist D, Jeppesen U, Andersen M, Garcia Rodriguez LA, Hallas J, Sindrup SH. Statins and risk of polyneuropathy: a case-control study. Neurology 2002; 58(9):1333-7.

31. Felton CV, Crook D, Davies MJ, Oliver MF. Relation of plaque lipid composition and morphology to the stability of human aortic plaques. Arterioscler Thromb Vas Biol. 1997;17:1337-45.

32. Wu DI, Liu J, Pang X, et al. Palmitic acid exerts pro-inflammatory effects on vascular smooth muscle cells by inducing the expression of C-reactive protein, inducible nitric oxide synthase and tumor necrosis factor. Int J Molecular Med. 2014;34:1706-12.

Chapter 14
Diet-induced muscle rot

The most obvious reason why muscles degenerate and become weak is due to a lack of exercise, which is absolutely true. Even if you eat a healthy diet, get enough sleep, and are not too stressed out, you can still lose muscle size and strength, which is why we should all exercise. This is especially true to maintain muscle mass as we age; and we know that muscle strength can be improved when older adults engage in a regular exercise program (1). This is very important because we know that greater muscle mass correlates with greater longevity (2).

Even the Centers for Disease Control has an e-book that focuses on the need for seniors to engage in strength training (3). Although this is true about exercise, we all have to face the fact that very few 80-90 year-old men are able to maintain the muscle tone of their youth. This is because the inflammaging process leads to the gradual loss of muscle mass no matter what we do. Despite this fact, it is possible to maintain adequate muscle mass till our final breath so we can enjoy our lives to the fullest.

Not surprisingly, the typical sedentary individual is not especially careful with his/her diet, so eating a pro-inflammatory diet serves to compound the problem of living a sedentary lifestyle. The outcome is the gradual or rapid progression towards obesity and the metabolic syndrome, which are associated with a rotting pro-inflammatory state within skeletal muscles (4), which is then made worse by the inflammaging process. So, if you want to successfully engage in physical activities as you move through your senior citizen years (60 and older), you need to achieve and maintain a DeFlamed state. Or, if you merely want to keep up with your kids, grandchildren, and even great grandchildren, you need to achieve and maintain a DeFlamed state.

The loss of muscle mass during the aging process typically becomes especially noticeable after the age of 60. The scientific term for muscle loss during aging is "sarcopenia of aging." The term "sarco" is derived from the term sarcoplasm, which essentially means the contents of a muscle cell, including the muscle fibers. The term "penia" means smaller, a deficiency, or a loss. Not surprisingly, the aging process involves the gradual increase in circulating pro-inflammatory cytokine levels, which in part accounts for the term inflammaging. And it is these cytokines that promote the gradual loss of muscle mass (5,6).

In addition to inflammaging, skeletal muscle loss is also accelerated in obese individuals (7). This is an exceptionally important issue to consider. Recall that 40% of adult Americans are obese and at least another 30% are overweight and moving towards obesity. As you read in Chapter 10, obesity is a rotting inflammatory state. In the context of skeletal muscle mass and health, the inflammatory chemistry of obesity leads to a progressive loss of muscle mass and function (7).

Before we discuss the pro-inflammatory changes that occur in skeletal muscle, we will first go over some basic musculoskeletal anatomy. Figure 1 illustrates the relationship among the muscle, tendons, and bones that make up the joint complex. The joint itself is a connection between two bones where movement occurs. In order for movement to occur, muscle(s), called prime movers, must contract. When these muscles contract, they exert a pulling force on their tendons that are inserted into bones, which allows for joint movement to occur. Notice very close to the joint itself a smaller muscle, which is referred to as a stabilizer.

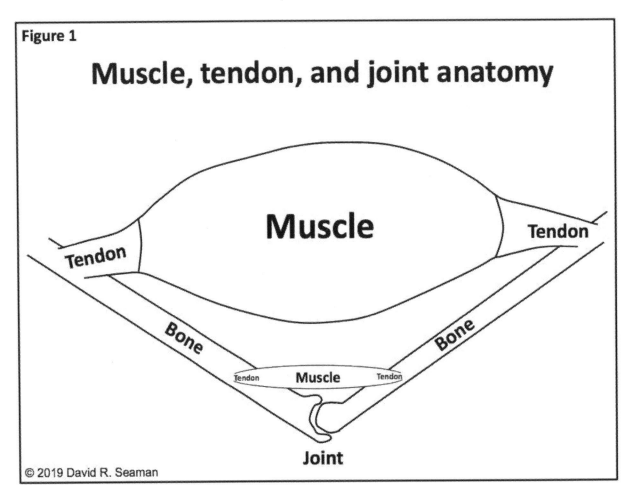

Most any healthcare professional who provides exercise recommendations will focus on improving the function of both stabilizers and prime movers. The term "core stability" is a common term and it typically refers to abdominal and low back muscles; however, joint stability is needed to prevent injury in any joint that is engage in mild to aggressive movements.

When people think about nutritional support for musculoskeletal tissues, they think calcium for bone, glucosamine/chondroitin for joints, and amino acids for muscles. While this is true, focusing on what musculoskeletal tissues need is NOT the proper DeFlame way to look at nutrition for musculoskeletal health. Instead, the DeFlame approach is to focus on what muscles, tendons, joints, and bones do NOT need and what causes them to degenerate and become painful and dysfunctional, and then consider what additional nutritional support measures may be useful.

It turns out that sedentary living and a pro-inflammatory diet are the two key factors that cause muscles to rot and become painful and dysfunctional. While amino acids are good for muscles, and calcium is good for bones, and glucosamine/chondroitin is good for joints, these nutrients are essentially useless if the "dietary flame" is too fierce, AND for most people the dietary flame is too fierce, especially when considered over the span of a lifetime. The remainder of this chapter will focus on how a pro-inflammatory diet leads to muscle degeneration, pain, and weakness, i.e., muscle rotting.

Fat accumulation in skeletal muscle (lipotoxicity)

As discussed in the previous chapter, part of the atherosclerotic process in arteries involves the accumulation of lipid, also known as fat. The term "lipid deposition in arteries" is synonymous with atherosclerosis, which is caused by the inflammatory state of the metabolic syndrome, diabetes, and/or obesity. If it is true that muscle degeneration is similar to atherosclerosis, as mentioned in Chapter 13, then we should also see evidence of lipid deposition in skeletal muscle in relation to the inflammatory states of the metabolic syndrome, diabetes, and/or obesity. In fact, this is the case and the subject has been studied in great detail (8-13).

Triglycerides are measured in a standard blood test. A triglyceride is a fat that contains a "backbone" called glycerol, to which three fatty acids are attached. Figure 2 is the least complicated way to accurately visualize a triglyceride. You can do an internet search for additional images of a triglyceride.

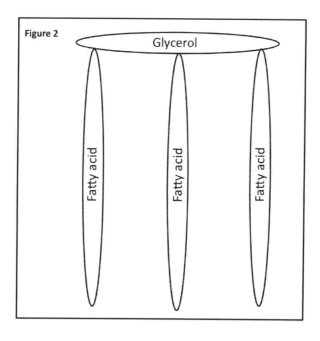

Triglycerides represent the body's storage form of fat, which can be used as energy when the time arises. No matter how lean or fat one is, we all have triglycerides in circulation. Additionally, triglycerides normally accumulate into what is called a lipid droplet in the healthy muscles of trained individuals. Lipid is synonymous with fat. In healthy individuals, muscles use the stored fat in lipid droplets as a source of ATP (energy) production for muscular/physical activities. In contrast with healthy individuals, fat accumulation in the muscles of overweight or obese people with the metabolic syndrome and diabetes is very different and reflects a rotting process. This is because the body is forced to store an excessive amount of fat in two ways.

First, there can be up to a 6-fold excess of triglyceride content in the skeletal muscle of patients with type 2 diabetes (9). This 6-fold excess of triglycerides accumulates over time as people gain body fat, become obese, and then develop the metabolic syndrome, and eventually diabetes.

Second, in addition to the excess of triglycerides, skeletal muscles of these individuals also accumulate abnormal fats called ceramide and diglyceride, which are associated with muscle inflammation and degeneration (10,11,13). Lipotoxicity is the term used to describe this type of abnormal fat accumulation that occurs with obesity.

Recall from Chapter 12 that a saturated fatty acid called palmitic acid or palmitate is the precursor for ceramide. This suggests that palmitic acid is a dangerous fatty acid, but this is not the case unless it is produced in excess. In fact, palmitic acid normally makes up 20-30% of all the saturated fatty acids in the human body (14). Additionally, up to 30% of breast milk fat is palmitic acid, demonstrating that it is an important calorie source for newborns (14). In short, palmitic acid is never a problem for the human body until it is produced in excess, which does occur in obesity, the metabolic syndrome and type 2 diabetes, and this is caused by the overconsumption of refined sugar and flour calories.

Recall from Chapters 6 and 10 that 40% of the average American's dietary calories comes from refined sugar and flour, which raises blood glucose levels. Liver and fat cells convert the excess glucose into an excess of palmitic acid (14,15). Some of the excess palmitic acid is incorporated into triglycerides, while the remainder circulates in the blood stream as palmitic acid, some of which enters skeletal muscle and is converted into ceramide, causing lipotoxicity (12,14,15)). As stated in Chapter 12, the accumulation of ceramide in skeletal muscle correlates directly to hyperinsulinemia and insulin resistance (15,16).

Additionally, the palmitic acid that is not converted into ceramide is a driver of chronic inflammation. Excess palmitic acid stimulates muscle cells to produce pro-inflammatory prostaglandin E2 (17), and also stimulates immune cells to release pro-inflammatory cytokines (18).

Figure 3 illustrates a normal DeFlamed muscle compared to an inflamed lipotoxic rotting muscle. The normal muscle contains a normal amount of lipid droplets that contain triglycerides. In contrast, the lipotoxic rotting muscle contains an excess of triglycerides, palmitic acid, as well as the abnormal diglycerides and ceramides. Because 70% of the adult US population is overweight or obese, this means that the majority of US adults are moving in the direction of developing muscle rot.

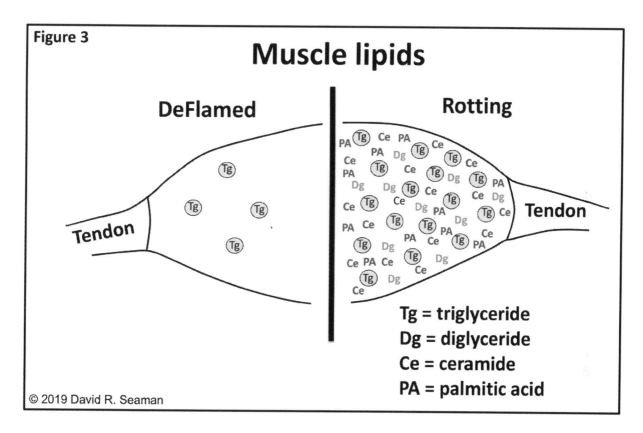

Here is a way you can get an idea if you have a lipotoxic problem in your muscles. You will need to look at your most recent blood test if you have one. If your fasting triglycerides are below 90 mg/dL, you are normal and have no issue with lipotoxicity. A fasting triglyceride level above 90 mg/dL is pro-inflammatory. If your fasting triglycerides are above 150 mg/dL, this is a marker for the metabolic syndrome, which is associated with lipotoxicity. This means that as people eat a pro-inflammatory diet and gradually increase their fasting triglyceride levels from 90 mg/dL to above 150 mg/dL, this represents a gradual march toward ceramide accumulation and thus, lipotoxicity.

In addition to accumulating in skeletal muscle, ceramide and diglycerides accumulate in multiple organs, the most notable being the liver, heart, and kidneys (13). Lipotoxicity, in its full manifestation, is estimated to affect approximately 25% of the adult US population (13). The accumulation of triglycerides, ceramide and diglycerides in skeletal muscle correlates with insulin resistance in skeletal muscle, which prevents skeletal muscle from properly taking up glucose from the blood stream, which allows for blood glucose levels to progressively rise (11,13).

Before moving to the next section, take another look at Figure 3. If you are lipotoxic it is important to understand that your rotting muscles will never function as they once did when you were young unless you get rid of the lipotoxic state. This will require you to DeFlame your diet and body, which is a straight-forward process that was briefly described early in this book in Chapter 1. For more detailed information, I urge you to read two of my other books, those being *The DeFlame Diet* and *Weight Loss Secrets You Need To Know*.

Energy deficiency in rotting muscles

Fat is supposed to be stored within fat cells in the skin, which is called subcutaneous fat. This is normal – even lean athletes have subcutaneous fat. As discussed in the previous section, it is NOT normal to store excess triglycerides, diglycerides, and ceramide in visceral organs and skeletal muscle. As these fats are progressively stored in skeletal muscle, there is an associated decrease in the ability of these lipotoxic muscles to utilize fat as a source of energy.

Energy production occurs in all cells of the body. This includes immune cells and the cells in all musculoskeletal structures and all visceral organs. Mitochondria are the specialized structures found in all cells that are responsible for energy production. Only red blood cells are able to create energy without mitochondria.

Mitochondria contain an energy-producing pathway called the Kreb's Cycle. A substance called acetyl-CoA enters the Kreb's Cycle and is broken down to create a cell energy molecule called adenosine triphosphate (ATP) that drives most bodily functions. We cannot eat acetyl-CoA; rather, our bodies make it from sugar, fats, and ketones. The synthesis of acetyl-CoA and the production of ATP work seamlessly until people start to eat excess calories. About 35% of the US population is overweight and another 35% is obese, which means that most Americans eat too many calories and either have already compromised, or will eventually compromise, their mitochondria.

As stated previously, almost 60% of the calories consumed by Americans come from refined sugar (20%), flour (20%), and oils (20%). The excess calories from all of these sources get stored as fat, and eventually leads to lipotoxicity as described above. Another problem develops due to an excess of refined sugar and flour consumption. The overconsumption of sugar and flour calories massively raises glucose entry into skeletal muscle and reduces the ability of muscle mitochondria to utilize fat for energy (19). This happens in just four weeks in normal individuals when they are given an additional 400 calories from sugar per day (19). Not surprisingly, this inability to utilize fat becomes worse and progresses over time.

In addition to mitochondria losing their ability to effectively burn fat for energy, there is a gradual and substantial reduction in the total population of mitochondria in skeletal muscle as chronic inflammation progresses over time (See Figure 3). This happens gradually as one puts on body fat weight, becomes obese, and develops the metabolic syndrome and then, type 2 diabetes (20). Additionally, the accumulation of ceramide in skeletal muscle, which was discussed in the previous section, participates in compromising mitochondria (15).

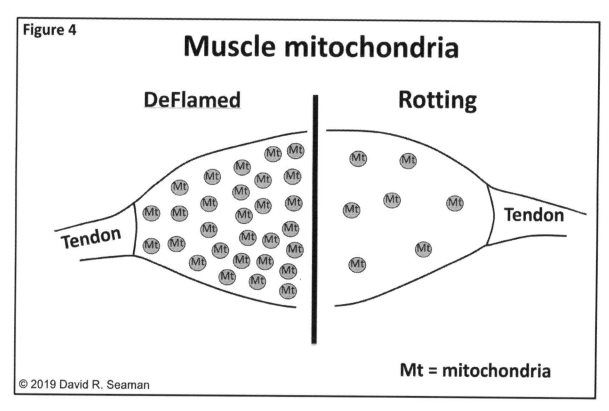

Muscle mitochondria

DeFlamed | **Rotting**

Tendon | Tendon

Mt = mitochondria

© 2019 David R. Seaman

At this point in this chapter, you should be impressed by the dramatic changes that occur in skeletal muscle in people who overeat refined carbohydrates and move toward developing obesity and insulin resistance. Imagine trying to move around or exercise with muscles that are lipotoxic and deficient in mitochondria; it is extremely difficult. People with such degenerated and rotting muscles feel weak and fatigued, and so they lack the motivation to exercise even though they know they should.

The first step for people in this situation is to DeFlame their diets, which can reduce chronic inflammation and improve muscle function, and reduce the feelings of weakness, fatigue, and depression. This allows people to feel better and become motivated to be more physically active. DeFlaming the diet will also help to normalize the immune profile and regenerative capacity of muscles that have been rendered lipotoxic and deficient in mitochondria.

Immune activity in normal vs rotting muscles

Few people think about the fact that muscles contain immune cells. One scientist remarked that, "immune cells are a long-overlooked component of healthy skeletal muscle" (21). For perspective, consider that our total blood supply contains approximately 4×10^{11} immune cells, whereas total muscle contains 4×10^{10} immune cells (21). As with the artery wall and body fat, the immune cell population in skeletal muscle can become pro-inflammatory, which is problematic, as skeletal muscles represent the largest organ in the human body. The last thing we need is for the immune cell population in the largest body organ to become pro-inflammatory, which is exactly what happens when people become obese and hyperglycemic and leads to the degeneration of skeletal muscle.

The weight gain process described in Chapter 10 is known to be associated with a shift from anti-inflammatory to pro-inflammatory immune cells in multiple tissues, including adipose tissue, blood vessels, pancreas, liver, and skeletal muscle (17,22-24). Figure 1 in Chapter 10 illustrates how anti-inflammatory immune cells are replaced by pro-inflammatory immune cells as one moves from being lean to obese. A similar shift occurs in muscles.

The most abundant immune cells in muscle are macrophages (21). M2 macrophages are anti-inflammatory and promote muscle proliferation and repair (25), so we want them there. In contrast, we don't want excess M1 macrophages because they are pro-inflammatory and cause tissue damage and prevent muscle repair (25). Figure 5 illustrates the pro-inflammatory macrophage shift that occurs in rotting muscles of obese individuals (17,26).

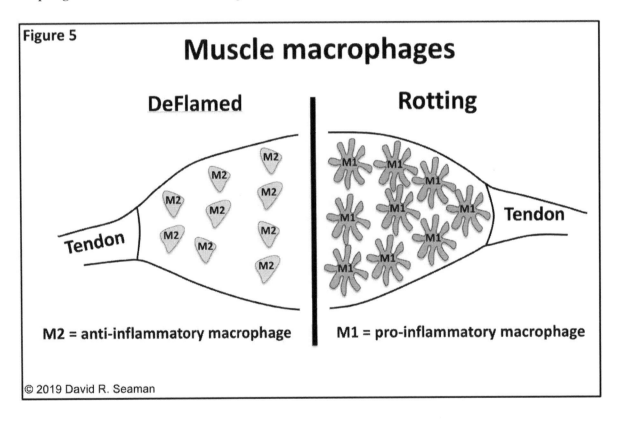

At this point in this chapter, if you are overweight or obese, you should be able to picture your muscles filling up with pro-inflammatory immune cells and lipotoxic fats, with a simultaneous deficiency in energy-producing mitochondria. This is clearly not something anyone needs and is a sign of insulin resistance, which is the hallmark sign of the metabolic syndrome and type 2 diabetes. If instead you are lean and healthy, your goal should be to never let your muscles flame up in this fashion.

As the pro-inflammatory state emerges in the body, not only immune cells participate in releasing pro-inflammatory prostaglandins and cytokines. It turns out that even muscles in these people begin to release pro-inflammatory cytokines (17,24). In fact (24):

> "Numerous studies have demonstrated an increase in inflammatory markers in skeletal muscle in people with obesity and diabetes. This includes activation of pro-inflammatory pathways within muscle cells themselves."

As stated in a previous section, when muscle cells are exposed to excess palmitic acid that does not get converted into ceramide, they release pro-inflammatory prostaglandin E2 (17). When exposed to endotoxin, which circulates in excess in people who are obese and insulin resistant, muscle cells release pro-inflammatory cytokines just like immune cells (17). This means that muscle cells can take on some of the behaviors of immune cells when we overeat pro-inflammatory calories, which leads to their own degradation.

Muscle regeneration is reduced by chronic inflammation
The only way to build muscle is to exercise and the only way to prevent muscle atrophy is to exercise. Essentially everyone understands this fact. One way to load muscles is with body weight, such as with pull-ups, push-ups, and lunges, to stimulate muscle growth. Another way is to also lift weights to increase the load placed on the exercising muscle(s), which is what most exercisers do, either at home or in the gym.

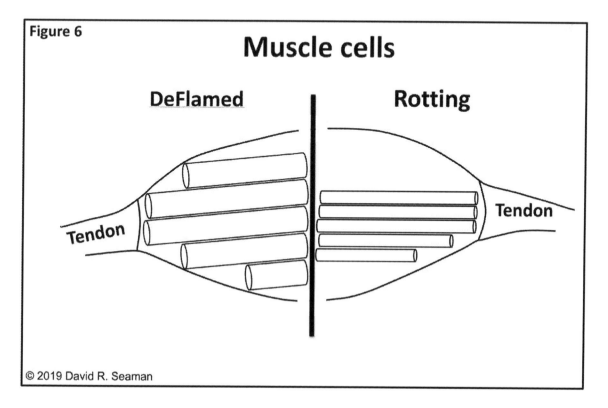

Virtually everyone knows that you can build muscle by exercising it, but very few people understand how this works in normal individuals or why it works much less efficiently in the inflamed population. To understand how muscle-building works, we need to understand the basic anatomy of a muscle. Figure 1 in this chapter illustrates the joint complex and the relationship among muscles, tendons, bones and a joint. Figure 6 illustrates muscle cell size in normal DeFlamed individuals compared to the atrophied muscle cells in the inflamed and rotting population. Not surprisingly, muscle cells are what make up the bulk of muscle tissue. A muscle cell is a long cylindrical tube. Only 5 muscle cells are illustrated for the purpose of showing the size differences. In real life, for example, we have over 200,000 muscle cells in the biceps muscle in the upper arm alone.

For many years, scientists have known that there are approximately the same amount of muscle cells in bodybuilders versus non-exercisers who were the same age (27). Additionally, it was discovered that young men (20 years old) and old men (80 years old) have the same amount of muscle cells. The biceps muscles of young men had 253,000 muscle cells, while the old men had 234,000 (28). This means that the difference in muscle mass appearance is primarily due to the size of muscle fibers, which grow bigger when exposed to an adequate load.

While certain people appear to have the ability to increase muscle cell size more easily than others, this should not lead to the belief that others are doomed to atrophy. This only means that the average person can modestly increase muscle cell size, or at least prevent atrophy, with regular exercise. It is also very important to create a DeFlamed state within the body because chronic inflammation causes muscle cells to atrophy, as illustrated in Figure 6 and 7.

Notice in Figure 7 that pro-inflammatory endotoxin enters into muscle cells and promotes the rotting process. It should not come as a surprise to you that muscle regeneration and muscle building processes involve muscle protein synthesis; this is why exercisers and body builders consume protein powders. Endotoxin, which circulates in excess in obese and insulin resistant individuals, enters skeletal muscle and lowers protein synthesis (17).

There is another reason why chronic inflammation leads to muscle atrophy and weakness, which is generally not-so-well-known and involves the presence of muscle stem cells. The term stem cell has become very popular and well known in recent years; however, it is only discussed in the context of using stem cells as treatments for various diseases. The topic is never discussed in the context of our skeletal muscles that contain readily available stem cells throughout our lifetime, which can be activated by exercise to help maintain adequate muscle mass throughout our lifetime.

Muscle stem cells are called satellite cells, which lie in close approximation to muscle cells. Satellite cells are needed to regenerate and heal muscle after injury or exercise. Notice in Figure 7 the abundance of satellite cells in the normal muscle and the reduced amount in the inflamed muscle.

Notice also that there are far less mitochondria in the inflamed (rotting) muscle, which means less energy production.

Figure 4 illustrated muscle mitochondria without including muscle cells so you could get a general appreciation of the differences between normal and inflamed muscles. In Figure 7, you can see that mitochondria are found inside muscle cells.

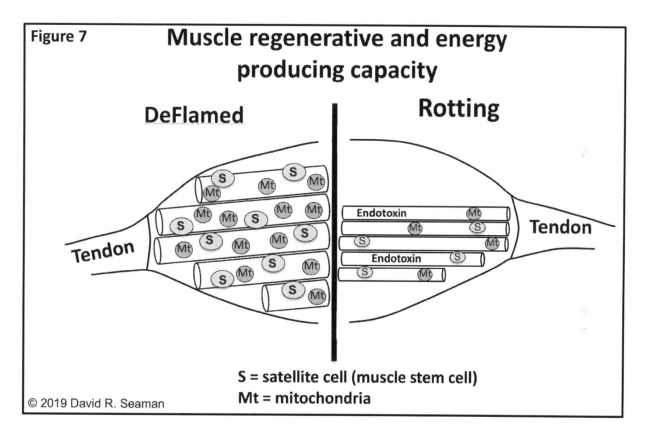

Before discussing how satellite cells work, it is important to understand why it is that exercisers never heavily load the same muscles day after day. The reason is because heavily loading muscles during exercise is a mildly injurious event that requires healing/repair to occur before another bout of heavy loading. In the context of muscle function, when the term load is used it just refers to the weight a muscle is trying to move, rather than compressive forces or loads that joints, spinal discs, and bone deal with, or tensile forces/loads that tendons deal with.

Following muscle injury, be it an accident or a heavy exercise bout, satellite cells, which lie adjacent to muscle cells, are activated and then proliferate and differentiate to form new muscle cells that grow and replace damaged muscle cells (29). This means that proper exercise (muscle loading to your fitness and tolerance level) will help muscle cells grow bigger and activate satellite cells to replace damaged muscle cells. Unfortunately, this process is compromised in obese and insulin resistant individuals. Figure 6 illustrates that muscle cells are smaller (atrophied) in these people and they have less satellite cells compared to the exercising population. Here is what scientists say about this (29):

> "Obesity and nutrient overload would be expected to provide unfavorable conditions for maintenance of quiescent satellite cells or for proliferation after acute injury."

When scientists say "nutrient overload" they are referring to high glucose levels (glucotoxicity) that compromise muscle function and the lipotoxic rotting process that develops as people moved toward obesity. In other words, glucotoxicity and lipotoxicity inhibit satellite cells. Pro-inflammatory immune activity also inhibits satellite cell activity.

Recall from the vitamin D and obesity chapters that T-regulatory cells (T-reg cells) were discussed. These are anti-inflammatory immune cells and they are depressed in the obese population and in those who are vitamin D deficient. It turns out that anti-inflammatory T-reg cells are very important for muscle regeneration because they promote satellite cell proliferation (30). In other words, a pro-inflammatory state will prevent T-reg cells from promoting satellite cell proliferation and lead to a loss of muscle mass.

To support normal satellite cell function, we simply need to DeFlame the body with nutrition and exercise at a load level that fits our fitness level. It need not be made any more complicated than that.

Summary of the inflammatory and degenerative changes in skeletal muscle
If you were to ask me for the most simplified explanation to factually describe the inflamed muscles of obese and insulin resistant people, this is what I would tell you:

> People who overeat and become insulin resistant have muscles that can be likened to "moveable sacks of inflammation that are fatigued, weak, and hurting most of the time."

If I was to tell you that and you were to ask me to explain it to you in more detail – then I would be telling you what is in this book. Most people are unaware of the information in this chapter about how muscles degenerate and flame up. I did not know all of this information until I wrote this chapter, which I tried to write in a fashion that can be understood by people without a science background. However, that does not mean that every bit of information will make complete sense to you the first time you read it. This should not stop you from understanding the information in this chapter.

Figure 8 includes all the rotting pro-inflammatory changes discussed in this chapter. A DeFlamed muscle has normal muscle cells, fat stores, mitochondria, satellite cells, immune cells, and no endotoxin. A goal for us all should be to have DeFlamed muscles, which would allow us to engage in whatever activities we desire.

In contrast, the absolute enemy of a healthy active life are inflamed, obese, and insulin resistant muscles, which have 1) atrophied muscle cells that are weak and easily fatigable, 2) lipotoxic fatty infiltration (excess ceramide, diglycerides, and triglycerides), 3) reduced mitochondria (less energy production), 4) reduced muscle-regenerating satellite cells, 5) an excess of pro-inflammatory immune cells, and 6) muscles cells that are compromised by endotoxin.

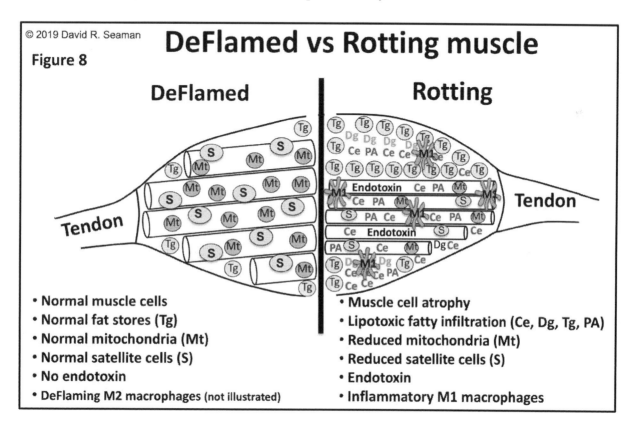

People with rotting muscles complain of soreness, fatigue, weakness, and exercise intolerance (31). Unfortunately, these people often suffer from a treatment that adds more symptoms. Most obese and diabetic patients with rotting muscles are also taking statin drugs, which were discussed in the previous chapter. Recall that many people who take statins suffer from side effects that included muscle pain, fatigue, memory loss, cognitive defects, irritability and aggression, and neuropathies (32-35).

It should not be a surprise to you that many people with rotting muscles feel essentially helpless and hopeless, so they choose not to take action. But you should not lose hope if this is you. I know many people who have pulled themselves out of the inflammatory abyss of body rot and now are enjoying their lives once again.

What should you do?

The picture painted in this chapter is hopefully scary enough to motivate you to never become obese and chronically inflamed. However, if you have reached the state of chronic inflammation illustrated in Figure 8, there are steps you can take.

1. Even though you may feel hopeless and helpless, you can reverse your situation; many, many people have done it. In other words, you are NOT helpless and you can certainly have hope. So you must have hope and this hope must be matched by proper action.

2. You need to embrace the DeFlame mindset, whether you choose to be a vegan, omnivore, or carnivore, as indicated in Chapters 1 and 12 of this book and in *The DeFlame Diet* book. Focus on substantially reducing your calories from pro-inflammatory foods and increasing your consumption of anti-inflammatory foods, and make sure you drop your total calorie intake so you can burn stored up excess body fat.

3. You must track your inflammatory markers as outlined in Chapter 3 of this book and in *The DeFlame Diet* book. This will keep your mind on track so that you are focused on multiple DeFlaming goals. The mind likes nothing better than specific goals to pursue.

4. You must develop the proper eating mindset and understand that we live in an obesogenic environment that pushes all of us to overeat. These topics are discussed in great detail in my book, *Weight Loss Secrets You Need To Know*.

5. You must engage in physical activities. Walking is better than nothing at all. When you can do this, walk as briskly as you can, which is much better than just casually strolling along. You must also engage in muscle loading (body weight exercises or weight lifting) to stimulate muscle cell growth. This should always be done based on your level of exercise tolerance. If you are not fit at all, you should never compare yourself to a fit person who can exercise for an hour straight. In short, it is very important to gradually load your muscles so you can avoid injury.

6. There are some supplements that are very beneficial to muscle mitochondria, the most notable and well known is coenzyme Q10 (CoQ10). There are three primary functions of CoQ10, which include 1) ATP synthesis by virtue of supporting mitochondria, 2) free radical modulation, and 3) the regulation of skeletal muscle gene expression (31). An example of skeletal muscle regulation was identified in 70 year-old men who were scheduled for hip replacement surgery.

For 25-30 days before surgery, the men either received 300 mg of CoQ10 per day or a placebo. At the time of surgery, samples of muscles from the thigh were taken from the same region, and gene and protein expression patterns and muscle fiber type profiles were compared between placebo and CoQ10-treated subjects. A shift in muscle fiber types towards the profiles of young people was observed in the subjects treated with CoQ10 (36).

My impression is that CoQ10 supplementation is advisable once we reach 30-40 years of age. I do not think we need to take 300 mg per day. As long as we are DeFlaming, 100 mg per day seems appropriate. Dr. Frederick Crane, the scientist who discovered CoQ10, explains that 100 mg per day will double the circulating blood level of CoQ10 in a clinically significant fashion (37). Other than CoQ10, supplementation should be viewed in the context of inflammation reduction as described in Chapter 9.

These six steps are easy to understand and implement. The most difficult hurdle to overcome for most people when starting the DeFlaming process is replacing overeating and sedentary living with new anti-inflammatory habits. Start the DeFlaming process at whatever level suits your mind and body and most importantly, commit to achieving normal inflammatory markers and maintaining them for the remainder of your life. You may not believe it, but most people start to feel better within the first week.

References
1. Sequin R, Nelson ME. The benefits of strength training for older adults. Am J Prev Med. 2003;25(3 Suppl 2):141-9.
2. Srikanthan P, Karlamangla AS. Muscle mass index as a predictor of longevity in older adults. Am J Med. 2014;127:547-53.
3. https://www.cdc.gov/physicalactivity/downloads/growing_stronger.pdf
4. Wu H, Ballantyne CM. Skeletal muscle inflammation and insulin resistance in obesity. J Clin Invest. 2017;127:43-54.
5. Dalle S, Rossmeislova L, Koppo K. The role of inflammation in age-related sarcopenia. Front Physiol. 2017;8: Article 1045.
6. Fan J, Kou X, Yang Y, Chen N. MicroRNA-regulated proinflammatory cytokines in sarcopenia. Mediators Inflammation. 2016; Article ID 1428686.
7. Sinha I, Sakthivel D, Varon DE. Systemic regulators of skeletal muscle regeneration in obesity. Front Endocrinol. 2017;8:29.
8. He J, Watkins S, Kelley DE. Skeletal muscle lipid content and oxidative activity in relation to muscle fiber type in type 2 diabetes and obesity. Diabetes. 2001;50:817-23.
9. Schrauwen-Hinderling VB, Hesselink MK, Schrauwen P, Kooi ME. Intramyocellular lipid content in human skeletal muscle. Obesity. 2006;14:357-67.
10. Martins AR, Nachbar RT, Gorjao R, et al. Mechanisms underlying skeletal muscle insulin resistance induced by fatty acids: importance of the mitochondrial function. Lipids Health Dis. 2012;11:30.

11. Li Y, Xu S, Zhang X, et al. Skeletal intramyocellular lipid metabolism and insulin resistance. Biophys Rep. 2015;1:90-98.

12. Tumova J, Andel M, Trnka J. Excess of free fatty acids as a cause of metabolic dysfunction in skeletal muscle. Physiol Res. 2016;65:193-207.

13. Nishi H, Higashihara T, Inagi R. Lipotoxicity in kidney, heart, and skeletal muscle dysfunction. Nutrients. 2019;11:1664.

14. Carta G, Murru E, Banni S, Manca C. Palmitic acid: physiological role, metabolism and nutritional implications. Frontiers Physiol. 2017;8: Article 902.

15. Hansen ME, Tippetts TS, Anderson MC. Insulin increases ceramide synthesis in skeletal muscle. J Diabetes Res. 2014; Article ID: 765784.

16. Turpin SM, Lancaster GI, Darby I, Febbraio MA, Watt MJ. Apoptosis in skeletal myotubes is induced by ceramides and is positively related to insulin resistance. Am J Physiol Endocrinol Metab. 2006;291:E1341-50.

17. Pillon NJ, Bilan PJ, Fink LN, Klip A. Cross-talk between skeletal muscle and immune cells: muscle-derived mediators and metabolic implications. Am J Physiol Endocrinol Metab. 2013;304:E453-65.

18. Nicholas DA, Zhang K, Hung C, et al. Palmitic acid is a toll-like receptor 4 ligand that induces human dendritic cell secretion of IL-1beta. PLoS ONE 12(5): e0176793.

19. Sartor R, Jackson MJ, Squillace C, et al. Adaptive metabolic response to 4 weeks of sugar-sweetened beverage consumption in healthy, lightly active individuals and chronic high glucose availability in primary human myotubes. Eur J Nutr. 2013;52:937-48.

20. Ritov VB, Menshikova EV, He J, et al. Deficiency of subsarcolemmal mitochondria in obesity and type 2 diabetes. Diabetes. 2005;54:8-14.

21. Tidball JG. Regulation of muscle growth and regeneration by the immune system. Nat Rev Immunol. 2017;17:165-78.

22. Lumeng CN, Saltiel AR. Inflammatory links between obesity and metabolic disease. J Clin Invest. 2011;121:2111-117.

23. Wu H, Ballantyne CM. Skeletal muscle inflammation and insulin resistance in obesity. J Clin Invest. 2017;127:43-54.

24. Lee YS, Wollam J, Olefsky JM. An integrated view of immunometabolism. Cell. 2018;172:22-40.

25. Mills CD. M1 and M2 macrophages: oracles of health and disease. Crit Rev Immunol. 2012;32:463-88.

26. Samaan MC. The macrophage at the intersection of immunity and metabolism in obesity. Diabetol Metab Syndr. 2011;3(1):29.

27. MacDougall JD, Sale DG, Always SE, Sutton JR. Muscle fiber number in the biceps brachii in bodybuilders and control subjects. J Appl Physiol Respir Environ Exerc Physiol. 1984;57:1399-403.

28. Klein CS, Marsh GD, Petrella RJ, Rice CL. Muscle fiber number in the biceps brachii muscle of young and old men. Muscle Nerve. 2003;28:62-68.

29. Akhmedov D, Berdeaux R. The effects of obesity on skeletal muscle degeneration. Front Physiol. 2013;4:Article 371.

30. Deyhle MR, Hyldahl RD. The role of T lymphocytes in skeletal muscle repair from traumatic and contraction-induced injury. Front Physiol. 2018;9: Article 768.

31. Fujimaki S, Kuwabara T. Diabetes-induced dysfunction of mitochondria and stem cells in skeletal muscle and the nervous system. Int J Mol Sci. 2017;18:2147.

32. Golomb BA. Statin adverse effects: implications for the elderly. Geriatric Times. May/June 2004. http://www.geriatrictimes.com/g040618.html

33. Wagstaff LR, Mitton MW, Arvik BM, Doraiswamy PM. Statin-associated memory loss: analysis of 60 case reports and review of the literature. Pharmacotherapy 2003; 23(7):871-880.

34. Golomb BA, Kane T, Dimsdale JA (2004), Severe irritability associated with statin cholesterol-lowering drugs. QJM 97(4):229-235.

35. Gaist D, Jeppesen U, Andersen M, Garcia Rodriguez LA, Hallas J, Sindrup SH. Statins and risk of polyneuropathy: a case-control study. Neurology 2002; 58(9):1333-7.

36. Linnane AW et al. Human aging and global function of coenzyme Q10. Ann N Y Acad Sci. 2002; 959:396-411.

37. Crane FL. Biochemical functions of coenzyme Q10. J Am Coll Nutr 2001; 20(6):591-598

Chapter 15
Osteoarthritis: Diet-induced joint rot

As described in Chapter 14, our skeletal muscles contract, which causes movement to occur in our joints so that we can engage in all physical activities. Figure 1 is an illustration of the bottom half of a normal joint. At the ends of the two bones that make up the joint, there is a specialized type of cartilage called articular (joint) cartilage, which is able to withstand compressive loading due to its unique biochemical nature. This will be described in more detail later in this chapter. For now, it is important to understand that joint cartilage in a normal joint is approximately 70% water, making it exceptionally hydrated and essentially incompressible (1).

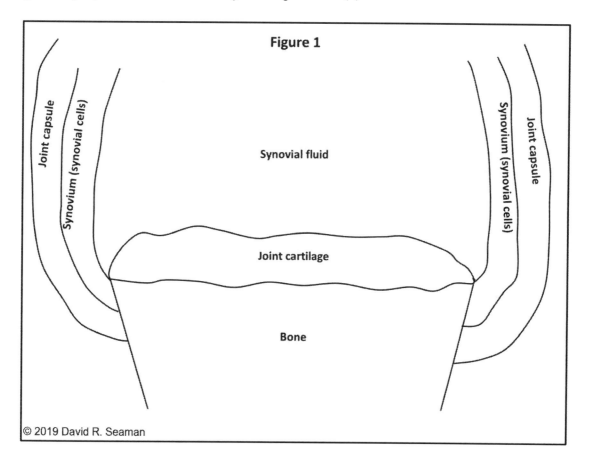

Notice in Figure 1 that a structure called the joint capsule surrounds the joint. Just inside the joint capsule is a structure called the synovium. Joint fluid is called synovial fluid, which is supposed to be produced throughout life by special cells in the synovium. Synovial fluid is especially slippery so movement can occur that is smooth and resistance-free within the allowable range of motion of a given joint.

Scientists use a term called the 'coefficient of friction' to describe the resistance to motion in a given system. It is somewhat difficult to conceptualize how minimal the friction is within human joints without the following examples. Picture in your mind that you are trying to move a rock across a piece of sandpaper – the coefficient of friction would be very high, which means there is a substantial resistance to movement. Now picture that same rock moving on ice – it has a much lower coefficient of friction and moves very easily without resistance. Even more slippery would be a piece of ice moving on ice. It turns out that the coefficient of friction in human joints is even more slippery than ice moving on ice.

With the above in mind, we should conceptualize a normal joint as being mostly a liquid structure. The joint cartilage is 70% water, which is lubricated by the liquid synovial fluid. Thus, a normal joint is essentially incompressible and exceptionally slippery (1), unless it is forced to deal with abnormally intense loads or if the structure of the remaining 30% of the joint cartilage is rendered pro-inflammatory and osteoarthritic due to poor dietary choices. Figure 2 illustrates a normal joint on the left and osteoarthritis on the right, with the most notable pro-inflammatory changes that occur in a joint with osteoarthritis (OA).

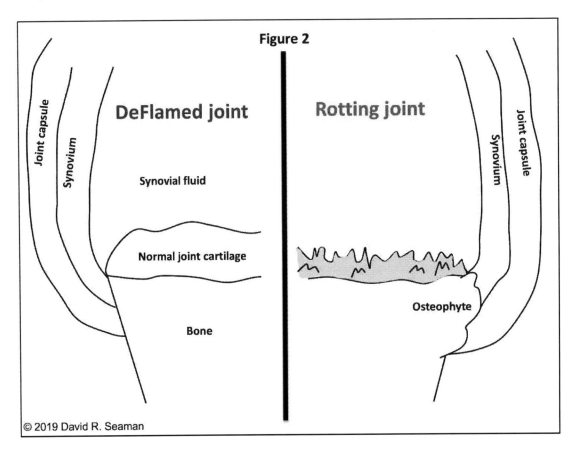

As you can see on the right side, osteoarthritic cartilage is degraded and there are pro-inflammatory boney outgrowths called osteophytes. Historically, these changes have been attributed to a wear and tear process, such that joint cartilage is believed to be damaged by a progressive grinding down type of phenomenon. We now know that this is not true at all. It is now known that multiple pro-inflammatory dietary factors work together in a cumulative fashion to cause osteoarthritis to develop, which can take many years to manifest as pain and then disability. Before discussing these dietary factors, the basics of normal joint anatomy and physiology will be briefly described.

Basic joint cartilage anatomy

The reason why so much of joint cartilage is water has to do with the specialized protein and carbohydrate content of the cartilage structure. Collagen is a protein and it is a component of joint cartilage, but it has little to do with why joint cartilage is exceptionally hydrated. The next three paragraphs will provide more details about how it is that joint cartilage is 70% water.

In addition to collagen, joint cartilage is also made of protein/carbohydrate structures called glycosaminoglycans, which are connected together to create a larger structure called a proteoglycan subunit. Individual proteoglycan subunits are connected together to create what is called a proteoglycan aggregate, which is also called aggrecan. Proteoglycans function like a like a sponge to suck up and retain water.

Figure 3. Proteoglycan aggregate (aggrecan)

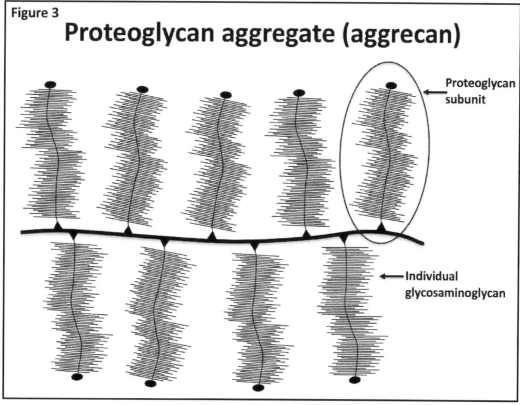

Figure 3 illustrates how aggrecan looks in joint cartilage. You can do an internet search for electron micrographs (pictures) of aggrecan in joint cartilage and spinal discs to see how similar this illustration is with the actual substance. Notice that nine proteoglycan subunits are connected to make aggrecan.

Glycosaminoglycans, and thus proteoglycans, contain an abundance of sulfate, which is negatively charged. In contrast, water is positively charged and is attracted to the negatively charged proteoglycans. You may have heard of nutritional supplements called glucosamine sulfate and chondroitin sulfate. These substances are also made by the body and become part of a proteoglycan, which is why they are recommended as supplements to support joint health. Again, it is the sulfate component that gives proteoglycans their negative charge to which water is attracted.

The word "imbibe" is often used when referring to drinking alcohol. "Imbibe" is also used in the scientific sense when referring to the taking up, or imbibition, of water by proteoglycans in joint cartilage, kind of like how a sponge imbibes water. While it can be a little hard to conceptualize, it turns out that a fully hydrated proteoglycan is about 1000 times larger compared to its dry weight size. This should also help you to understand how joint cartilage can consist of 70% water. Even though you may have never heard of proteoglycans before, you should now understand that it is our hydrated proteoglycans that allow for joint cartilage to withstand substantial compressive loading without injury.

How the human body makes collagen

Collagen is a structural protein and accounts for about a third of all the protein found in the human body. Without collagen our skin and musculoskeletal and visceral tissues would not have the structural appearance that we currently have.

The structure of collagen is that of a fiber, so not surprisingly, it is said that the various connective tissues in the body (joints, tendons, spinal discs, etc.) are made up of collagen fibers. These same tissues also contain proteoglycans, which will be discussed in more detail in the next section.

The primary cells in the human body that produce collagen are called fibroblasts and chondrocytes. In general, fibroblasts are found in skin (dermis), tendons, spinal discs, ligaments, and the fascia that surrounds muscles and visceral organs. In contrast, chondrocytes are found in joint cartilage and in the endplate area of the spinal disc (to be described in Chapter 17). Fibroblasts and chondrocytes require all of the essential nutrients that are required by all other cells in the body.

Collagen synthesis is rarely compromised. In fact, the opposite is true. The term fibrosis is used to describe an excess of connective tissue deposition. Most chronic diseases, such as cancer, heart disease, Alzheimer's disease, liver cirrhosis, rheumatoid arthritis, chronic pancreatitis, pulmonary (lung) fibrosis, and glomerulosclerosis (kidney disease) are referred to as chronic inflammatory fibroproliferative diseases, which involve the overproduction of connective tissue (2). This means that we want to create a DeFlamed state of body chemistry that prevents fibroproliferative activity.

In the context of specific nutrients, it is known that both magnesium and vitamin D regulate collagen metabolism to prevent inappropriate proliferation (3,4), as in the abovementioned diseases.

In my view, the nutritional focus for collagen should be preventing an excess of production, as discussed in the previous paragraph, and also protecting it after it is synthesized. The colorful pigments found in vegetation, called polyphenols, protect collagen from pro-inflammatory degradation (5,6), which means that a diet rich in vegetation should be a focus.

How the human body makes glycosaminoglycans and proteoglycans
As with collagen, the primary cells that produce glycosaminoglycans (GAGs) and proteoglycans (PGs) are fibroblasts and chondrocytes. The difference between collagen and GAGs/PGs is that collagen is a protein that is derived from amino acids while GAGs/PGs are derived from glucose and also contain some amino acids. Because the GAG/PG structure also contains amino acids, they are glycosAMINOglycans and PROTEOglycans.

The metabolic pathway that makes GAGs/PGs requires magnesium in most steps, which is partly why scientists explain that magnesium is a pivotal actor in connective tissue regulation (3). As stated in Chapter 9, there are more than 300 metabolic reactions in the body that require magnesium and many involve anti-inflammatory actions. ATP synthesis for energy also requires magnesium, as does GAG/PG synthesis. As stated in Chapter 9, the typical recommendation for magnesium supplementation is 400-1000 mg per day.

Osteoarthritis: diet-induced joint rot
While not everyone with joint pain has osteoarthritis, they still have many of the pro-inflammatory changes that occur with osteoarthritis, which makes it the ideal condition to study to better understand joint pain, joint inflammation, and joint degeneration, which I am referring to as joint rot so it can be properly conceptualized. The outcome of knowing this information should lead you to take the proper anti-inflammatory steps to protect your joints.

<u>Trauma misconception</u>
Most people with joint pain have not suffered from an obvious traumatic/injurious event that subsequently led to the development of osteoarthritis (OA). Despite this fact, chiropractors, physical therapists, and medical doctors continue to be trained to believe that joint trauma is the primary cause of osteoarthritis. However, research into the various causes of osteoarthritis demonstrates that only about 12% of all cases are caused by trauma (7).

Another fact that gets blurred about trauma-induced osteoarthritis is that between 20-50% of people with obvious joint trauma develop osteoarthritis. In other words, more than 50% of people who suffer obvious traumatic injuries do NOT develop OA (7).

The ankles and knees are the most commonly injured joints that develop osteoarthritis. What is generally not appreciated is the fact that trauma-induced OA is most common in young adults, not the older population, AND it is the older population that suffers primarily with osteoarthritis.

We know that more than 50% of post-traumatic OA recovers within 2-3 months (8). Pain that persists beyond 3 months suggests that chronic inflammation is the problem. After 6 months, post traumatic OA is absolutely considered an inflammatory condition (8). This may be due to the severity of the injury or the person who was injured was already "flaming" too much and unable to heal properly.

If osteoarthritis emerges without obvious trauma, which is the scenario for most people with osteoarthritis, it is most likely associated with the metabolic syndrome. This is most common in people over the age of 45 (9). In fact, scientists now believe that osteoarthritis is a part of the metabolic syndrome. In 2012, researchers stated (9):

> "In this review, we summarize the shared mechanisms of inflammation, oxidative stress, common metabolites and endothelial dysfunction that characterize the etiologies of OA and metabolic syndrome, and nominate OA as the fifth component of the metabolic syndrome."

Almost 60% of people with the metabolic syndrome have osteoarthritis (9). In the United States, approximately 20% of women and almost 25% of men between the ages of 40-49 have the metabolic syndrome (10). This rises to almost 35% of men and women between the ages of 50-59, and further increases to 45% among the population of 60 and older (10).

It should be understood that multiple pro-inflammatory factors can promote OA expression in people who do not suffer a traumatic injury. The metabolic syndrome is probably the biggest issue. Other pro-inflammatory factors will be discussed later in this chapter.

Wear and tear misconception
In the previous section, you learned that trauma is involved in only 12% of OA cases and this typically develops in young people after injury who do not heal within the typical 3-month window. While post-traumatic OA does occur in just 12% of the population, wear and tear osteoarthritis is something that NEVER occurs.

In this section, we will examine the wear and tear misconception, which remains the most common belief among healthcare professions about how OA develops. Indeed, the belief is that OA develops gradually over time due to wear and tear that is not associated with inflammation.
For many years, I have found this to be a surprising perception to maintain because since at least the early 1980s, scientists identified osteoarthritis to be an inflammatory state in joint tissue (11-14). Here is the title from a 2016 paper that tells the whole story in the title:

Robinson WH, et al. Low-grade inflammation as a key mediator of the pathogenesis of osteoarthritis. Nat Rev Rheumatol. 2016;12:580-92.

Due to the presence of chronic low-grade inflammation, joints gradually lose their ability to repair after normal compressive loading. Thus, OA should be properly conceptualized as a *wear and lack of repair* condition due to the presence of low-grade inflammation. This chapter will demonstrate how over time, our joints flame up, which eventually renders them less able to undergo the normal wear and repair processes that keeps joints functioning properly. Over many years, the wear and lack of repair leads to joint degradation that eventually becomes noticeable on x-ray, which is then misinterpreted to be caused by wear and tear.

This chapter will outline the many factors that participate in creating a pro-inflammatory state, which eventually prevent joints from repairing properly after normal activities. With this knowledge, you will understand what you should do to protect your joints to keep you active during your aging years.

Matrix metalloproteinases and joint cartilage degradation

Matrix metalloproteinases (MMPs) are enzymes that degrade connective tissue. They were initially discussed in Chapter 13 in the context of their involvement in atherosclerosis. It is important to understand what MMPs are because they degrade joint cartilage to cause the osteoarthritis changes that are seen on x-rays. These same enzymes degrade tendons to cause tendon pain called tendinopathy, and they also degrade the spinal disc which can lead to disc herniation.

When I went through school, the various connective tissue degrading enzymes were named based on the individual connective tissue type. For example, collagen-degrading enzymes were called collagenases. There are numerous types of collagen and so there are different types of collagenase enzymes that are more specific to the specific type of collagen. Proteoglycan-degrading enzymes should have been called proteoglycanases, but instead they were called stromelysins. Eventually scientists created a nomenclature system for all the various connective tissue degrading enzymes. As stated above, the various enzymes are called matrix metalloproteinases (MMPs), and they are numbered MMP-1, MMP-2 and so on. To date, almost 30 different MMPs have been identified.

There is no routine lab test to see if you have elevated MMP activity putting your joints and other tissues at risk. Fortunately, we have a way to indirectly identify if we suffer from elevated MMP activity. Scientists have identified that MMP activity is increased in people with the metabolic syndrome (15), which means we should be tracking the metabolic syndrome markers discussed previously in Chapters 3 and 12 and get them to normal levels so we can properly regulate MMP activity and prevent the development of OA.

To normalize MMP activity, my perception is that we should get our metabolic syndrome markers into the normal range, and additionally take the key supplements I discussed previously. It turns out that the common nutrients I think are valuable as supplements to help reduce inflammation in general, are also known to help regulate MMP activity, those being omega-3 fatty acids, vitamin D, magnesium, and polyphenols (16-21).

Insulin resistance and osteoarthritis

At this point in this book, insulin resistance has been discussed in adequate detail for you to understand that both the metabolic syndrome and type 2 diabetes are insulin resistance syndromes. You should now understand that insulin resistance is a pro-inflammatory state that is characterized by hyperglycemia, hyperlipemia, and hyperinsulinemia, which leads to an increase in the production of free radicals, cytokines and other pro-inflammatory chemicals. Not surprisingly, the metabolic syndrome is now viewed as a promoter of osteoarthritis (22), and as stated in the previous section, scientists have proposed that that OA is actually a component of the metabolic syndrome (9). Even worse, type 2 diabetes is an independent predictor for developing *severe* osteoarthritis (23). The people who believe that OA is a wear and tear condition never take these facts into consideration.

With the above information in mind, you should understand why it is that anti-inflammatory drugs can never properly control the inflammation and degradation of joint cartilage when it is caused by insulin resistance and its related pro-inflammatory chemistry. This is the same reason why just supplementing with glucosamine and chondroitin products is often unimpressive. Drugs and supplements for osteoarthritis cannot combat the body and joint inflammation created by the pro-inflammatory insulin resistant state. People need to reverse the metabolic syndrome and diabetes to stop the chronic flame that degrades their joints.

Again, the fact that people with the metabolic syndrome and type 2 diabetes are more likely to have OA speaks to the fact that OA is a wear and lack of repair condition. When we are flamed up, we simply do not have the wherewithal to heal properly after normal wear or with injury.

Advanced glycation end products (AGEs) and osteoarthritis

Anyone with an elevated blood glucose level is likely to have had their hemoglobin A1c (HbA1c) level checked. HBA1c is an AGE and is also called glycated hemoglobin, which means that hemoglobin has been excessively "sugared up."

Other tissues and substances can be glycated due to hyperglycemia; not just hemoglobin. As an example, LDL cholesterol can be glycated, which promotes the oxidation of LDL. In aging cartilage, high levels of AGEs called pentosidine, carboxymethyllysine and carboxyethyllysine, accumulate and create inflammation that promote osteoarthritis (24).

The chondrocytes that make collagen and proteoglycans for joint cartilage have receptors for AGEs. The presentation of AGEs to chondrocytes leads to the release of cytokines and the subsequent degradation of joint cartilage (25).

Practically speaking, the best way to identify how inappropriately glycated you may be is to measure HbA1c. It should be below 5.7%, which is normal. Anything above that indicates that you are over-glycated. I have seen people at 11%, which is very high and diagnostic for type 2 diabetes, reduce it back to normal within a few months by heavy dietary DeFlaming.

Recall from Chapter 2 that AGEs are found in animal products and are substantially increased when dry heat cooking methods are used. The degree to which such dietary AGEs cause osteoarthritis or any other condition in the absence of the metabolic syndrome or type 2 diabetes is not known.

C-reactive protein (CRP) and osteoarthritis
Multiple studies have confirmed that CRP levels are modestly elevated in OA patients compared to controls. Of greater clinical significance, in patients with OA, increased CRP levels have been associated with disease progression and clinical severity. Elevations of CRP are not only present in OA patients, but may help predict emergent OA (26).

Clearly, we want our CRP levels to be normal, and this means less than 1 mg/L. The blood test for CRP is readily available and inexpensive. CRP levels can readily return to normal with The DeFlame Diet along with getting adequate exercise and sleep.

Obesity and osteoarthritis
Not everyone who is obese will necessarily have the metabolic syndrome or diabetes. Overtime, most obese people will eventually develop insulin resistance; however, the obesity state of inflammation can exist to varying degrees without an associated manifestation of the metabolic syndrome or diabetes.

As outlined in Chapter 10, obesity is a pro-inflammatory cytokine state, involving an overproduction of IL-1, IL-6, and TNF, which is thought to be a promoter of osteoarthritis (27). With this in mind, as of the year 2005, scientists stated that (26), "there is compelling evidence that inflammatory cytokines such as IL-1, IL-6, and TNF disrupt cartilage homeostasis and help direct the progressive, MMP-mediated digestion of cartilage in OA."

Not only do the pro-inflammatory cytokines promote the degradation of collagen and proteoglycans, these same cytokines inhibit chondrocytes in joints from synthesizing adequate amounts of collagen and proteoglycans (27). There should be no doubt in your mind that we cannot "wear away" our joint cartilage; rather, it gets progressively digested or degraded away by the MMPs that do not get turned off properly due to chronic inflammation.

Free radicals promote osteoarthritis
When you read or hear about free radicals, my suggestion is to think about the information and image in Chapter 8 of this book. Free radicals are produced by all cells as part of normal

biochemistry and physiology. The problem is when the production exceeds that of free radical reduction. First, it is important to understand that hyperglycemia, hyperlipemia, and hyperinsulinemia of the metabolic syndrome and diabetes are associated with a generalized state of increased free radical production. Second, scientists have identified localized free radical excess in various diseases, including osteoarthritis (28,29). It turns out that a chronic pro-inflammatory diet causes chondrocytes to become pro-inflammatory and release cytokines, MMPs, and free radicals that degrade their own joint cartilage.

OA as a cardiovascular disease

At this point, you should realize that the same pro-inflammatory chemistry is found in the metabolic syndrome, diabetes, heart disease, and osteoarthritis. Recall that in Chapters 13 and 14, I explained how lipid (fat) deposition occurs in both atherosclerotic heart disease and in skeletal muscle in people who are obese and insulin resistant. The same lipid deposition process occurs in joints (30,31). Consider the title of this article, which describes this relationship:

> Gkretsi V, Simopoulou T, Tsezou A. Lipid metabolism and osteoarthritis: lessons from atherosclerosis. Prog Lipid Res. 2011;50:133-40.

In this article, the authors stated that lipid deposition in the joint is observed at the early stages of osteoarthritis (OA) before the occurrence of histological changes (31), which means microscopic changes. At this stage in the disease, there would be no symptoms and no identifiable changes on x-ray, MRI, or CAT scan. This means that joint anatomy can subtly change into a low-grade pathological state without any signs or symptoms, which is identical to how atherosclerotic heart disease develops. When the pathological state reaches a critical level in the knee, OA pain appears. In contrast, when the pathological state reaches a critical level in a coronary artery, a heart attack can occur. You can see why it is foolish to view OA as a wear and tear condition. Biochemically, OA is essentially heart disease of the joints.

Another commonality between OA and heart disease is LDL cholesterol. Recall from Chapter 12 and 13 that LDL cholesterol is an atherosclerosis driver in arteries *only* when it is oxidized, which is caused by hyperglycemia, hyperinsulinemia, and trans fats. A similar scenario holds true for joint cartilage. It turns out that circulating oxidized LDL gets into our joints and stimulates the cells in the synovium (macrophages, endothelial cells, and fibroblasts) to release pro-inflammatory cytokines and the metalloproteinases that degrade joint cartilage (32).

Omega-6 fatty acids and osteoarthritis

The omega-6 fatty acids we eat get incorporated into the cell membranes of our body cells, and this includes chondrocytes in joint cartilage (33-35). Recall from the free radical chapter in this book (Chapter 8):

We are supposed to consume a diet of less than a 4 to 1 ratio of omega-6 to omega-3 fatty acids in the diet, which is described in more detail in several chapters in *The DeFlame Diet* book (Chapters 18, 25, 26).

By 1991, researchers identified that normal, young cartilage has exceptionally low levels of omega-6 fatty acids, the most notable being arachidonic acid (34). This was found to be the case in young chickens, fetal calf, newborn pigs, rabbits, and humans. Young cartilage in all these species also had an unusually high level of an omega-9 fatty acid called mead acid. What is unique about mead acid is that is metabolically inactive, compared to arachidonic acid, which is highly inflammatory. Overtime as we age, arachidonic acid levels progressively increase and replace mead acid in joint cartilage. This is due to overeating grain-fed animals, deep-fried and packaged foods prepared with omega-6 oils, including those from corn, safflower, sunflower, cottonseed, soybeans, and peanuts. This means that these omega-6 foods change the normal structure of joint cartilage from one that is non-inflammatory to one that is pro-inflammatory.

By the time the average person reaches their 30s, their joint cartilage has already been transformed into a low-grade rotting inflammatory state, which is no longer able to withstand normal or aggressive loading patterns. The degree to which this happens varies from person to person, which means that the degree to which joint cartilage can wear and not repair also varies from person to person.

If you want to protect your joint cartilage from degeneration, you need to stop eating foods that are rich in omega-6 fatty acids. Otherwise, your joints will continue to load up on omega-6s and, sooner or later, the outcome will be chronic joint pain. Omega-3 supplements can help, but only if dietary omega-6 consumption is drastically lowered back to normal by eating anti-inflammatory foods.

Vitamin D and osteoarthritis

Imagine you read or heard somewhere that vitamin D helps osteoarthritis, so you start taking it. The chance that just taking vitamin D will be helpful is only likely if all of the above-mentioned drivers of OA are normal. In other words, vitamin D deficiency is just one of many risk factors that promotes osteoarthritis (36). As stated in Chapter 11, a reasonable vitamin D goal is to get your 25(OH)D level to 70 ng/mL.

Endotoxin and osteoarthritis

Endotoxin was first discussed in this book in the obesity section. It is derived from gram-negative bacteria. We all have a very small and tolerable amount of endotoxin in circulation, which increases with a pro-inflammatory diet, obesity and dental disease. Because endotoxin is such a small molecule, it can be delivered wherever blood and nutrients are delivered. In the case of this chapter, we are focusing on joints. Endotoxin can certainly get into the synovium and perhaps joint cartilage.

110

Both synovial cells and chondrocytes in joint tissues are known to produce inflammatory cytokines in response to an endotoxin challenge. This has led scientists to state that, "endotoxin could be considered a major hidden risk factor that provides a unifying mechanism to explain the association between obesity, metabolic syndrome and osteoarthritis" (37). In fact, one study suggested that endotoxin is a cause of tissue destruction and disintegration of joint cartilage in osteoarthritis (38).

The fact that circulating endotoxin is derived from the gut and mouth demonstrates that we should not load up on refined sugar, flour, and oils, which flame up the gut and mouth and lead to increased levels of circulating endotoxin, which can flame up our joints. More importantly, this demonstrates that focusing on trauma as the primary cause of osteoarthritis is shortsighted at best. It is far more accurate to view osteoarthritis as a state of chronic joint rot.

Summary

After reading the previous sections, it should be clear that osteoarthritis is a rotting process that is primarily caused by multiple factors related to a pro-inflammatory diet, namely hyperglycemia, advanced glycation end products (AGEs), obesity, excess free radicals (FRs), oxidized cholesterol (oxLDL), omega-6 fatty acids, and endotoxin. Figure 4 encapsulates these dietary factors in association with the visual image of joint cartilage degradation.

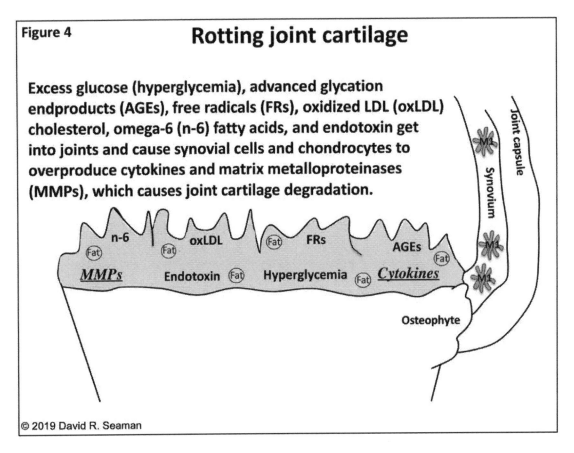

Figure 4

Rotting joint cartilage

Excess glucose (hyperglycemia), advanced glycation endproducts (AGEs), free radicals (FRs), oxidized LDL (oxLDL) cholesterol, omega-6 (n-6) fatty acids, and endotoxin get into joints and cause synovial cells and chondrocytes to overproduce cytokines and matrix metalloproteinases (MMPs), which causes joint cartilage degradation.

© 2019 David R. Seaman

Notice also in Figure 4 that excess immune cells (M1 macrophages) accumulate in the synovium. In a recent study, the researchers found that greater accumulation of M1 macrophages correlated with increased severity of osteoarthritis (39). Recall the pro-inflammatory immune shift that was described in the chapters on vitamin D, obesity, the metabolic syndrome, heart disease, and muscle degeneration. The same pro-inflammatory shift occurs in osteoarthritic joints (40).

Supplements that help joints
At this point in the chapter, it should be exceptionally clear that supplementation without modifying the dietary factors listed above will probably not deliver much pain relief. It is certainly possible to get relief, but if you don't, you will have to address the various pro-inflammatory dietary factors. And if you want to protect your joints and age gracefully, you should DeFlame the diet sooner rather than later.

My approach to supplementation has already been described in Chapter 9. This is a reasonable approach to supplementation for the general support of metabolism and inflammation reduction. In the next section, I will outline a few supplements that deserve special consideration for osteoarthritis.

Glucosamine and chondroitin sulfate
When glucosamine sulfate originally became popular in the 1980s or 90s, it was promoted by the marketeers as a cure for arthritis, even though there was no evidence indicating that it actually was a cure. Despite this fact, it became an exceptionally popular supplement, however, it eventually lost its luster in the patient-treatment world. This is because the placebo component of the treatment effect wore off. Here is what you need to know about glucosamine sulfate and chondroitin sulfate supplements…

Glucosamine is a precursor in the synthesis of glycosaminoglycans and proteoglycans. Chondroitin is a glycosaminoglycan. Both have been popular over the years as individual supplements and in combination.

In 2001, the results of a 3-year study with glucosamine sulfate (1500 mg/day) compared to placebo for knee OA pain was published in a famous British medical journal called the Lancet (41). The 106 subjects taking glucosamine sulfate had less pain and almost no loss of joint space, compared to the 106 subjects taking the placebo. The average age of the subjects was 60 years. This study was the first to scientifically demonstrate the benefit of glucosamine sulfate in osteoarthritis of the knee.

In 2006, an OA knee pain trial involving almost 1600 subjects compared glucosamine, chondroitin, glucosamine/chondroitin, Celebrex, and placebo (42). It was a double-blinded trial so none of the doctors or patients knew who was getting what treatment. The study lasted 24 weeks and the subjects' average age was 59 years. The outcomes were based on the severity of the OA; 1230 subjects had mild OA pain, while the remaining subjects' pain was rated as severe. In the mild pain group, there was no difference in pain reduction among the different treatments. However, in the severe pain group, the glucosamine/chondroitin had the best results and beat the medication (Celebrex) by 10%.

With the above outcomes in mind, you need to know that at least a 20% or greater reduction in pain was considered a successful outcome. With this in mind, I am the same age as the subjects in the above two glucosamine trials. My favorite physical activities include golf, surfing, bicycling, lifting weights, and doing yard work. If my back hurts at a 5/10 pain level (0 being pain-free and 10 being the worst pain imaginable), I would not be able to enjoy any of those activities. So, let's say I take glucosamine and my pain level drops to a 4/10. According to the scientific literature, I am a treatment success, however, I would still not be able to enjoy my favorite activities any more than when I was a 5/10. As a patient, I would view glucosamine to be a failure...even though, scientifically speaking, it was a success. In other words, most people with osteoarthritis need to do more than just take a glucosamine supplement.

In 2007, scientists published an article that described their research effort to discover patient markers that could identify why certain people with knee OA pain had success with glucosamine supplementation compared to those that did not (43). A key marker was body mass index (BMI). The study that demonstrated the best outcomes in terms of pain reduction and joint space protection involved subjects with an average age of 62 years with a BMI of about 25.7, which means they were just barely overweight (44). In other words, you are likely to have the best chance of being helped with glucosamine supplementation if you are not overweight. This outcome speaks to the primary focus of The DeFlame Diet, and that is getting body weight into the normal range.

Ginger
In 1992, researchers interviewed 56 people who had been taking powdered ginger to help reduce pains due to osteoarthritis, rheumatoid arthritis, or basic muscle and joint pain (45). Questionnaires were filled out to determine the utility of ginger. The results revealed that several individuals were able to reduce or eliminate their reliance on dangerous anti-inflammatory medications, with no other lifestyle changes other than taking ginger.

One subject was an 80 year-old woman with OA who took ginger for 3 years. During the first 6 months, she took 6 grams of ginger per day, and then reduced it to 2 grams for the remaining two and half years and was able to effectively control her pain. Ginger does not have any of the side effects of aspirin and other non-steroidal anti-inflammatory drugs (NSAIDs), which is great for everyone and especially great for the aged population. In short, ginger has many anti-inflammatory functions.

On a personal note, my youngest brother was a former catcher on his college baseball team, and he played against minor league ballplayers in summer leagues. He also excelled in many other sports – he was an exceptional amateur athlete. From years of catching, he developed significant pain in both knees. When he graduated and began working at a desk job, after sitting for periods of 1/2 hour or longer, it took him 10-12 steps to stand fully upright and walk with half the pain he had when sitting, and he was only in his 20's at the time. He began drinking ginger tea that was made from fresh ginger root, as well as taking ginger root capsules (4-6 grams/day). Within a month, the pain was gone, and he was able to get up from a seated position and could walk normally with no pain at all. It is important to understand that this is a common outcome for young, healthy people as long as their diet is not terribly pro-inflammatory. My brother was just 27 when he had this excellent response to ginger. Older and more inflamed people typically need to go to greater DeFlaming lengths to achieve a similar outcome. In the case of my brother who is now almost 50, he still follows his ginger regimen and the DeFlame approach to eating, and his knees remain pain free.

Magnesium

As stated earlier in this chapter, magnesium is involved with both collagen and proteoglycan synthesis (3). Magnesium also improves bone metabolism related to joint health, helps cartilage regeneration, and reduces inflammation (46). Not surprisingly, studies have been done to see if magnesium can help improve osteoarthritic joints. Scientists injected magnesium into the joints of rats with osteoarthritis, which lead to the improvement of new cartilage synthesis and inflammation reduction (47). This does not mean that supplementing with magnesium will restore joints to normal, but it does confirm the need to make sure you have adequate magnesium intake for normal joint cartilage function. In fact, scientists believe that magnesium supplementation is a promising supportive therapy for joint health and the treatment of osteoarthritis (48).

What you can do

The degree to which joint pain and osteoarthritis can be modulated varies from person to person. The time it takes for improvement to occur is also variable. The first key step is to DeFlame the diet and maintain normal body weight. This will immediately reduce the dietary drive that promotes osteoarthritis and all other debilitating conditions, such as depression, diabetes, heart disease, cancer, and Alzheimer's disease. The various supplements discussed above and in Chapter 9 can also be taken, with the goal in mind to reduce inflammatory markers back to normal.

References

1. Morrell KC, Hodge WA, Krebs DE, Mann RW. Corroboration of in vivo cartilage pressures with implications for synovial joint tribology and osteoarthritis causation. Proc Nat Acad Sci. 2005;102:14819-24.
2. Ross R. Atherosclerosis – an inflammatory disease. New Eng J Med. 1999;340:115-26.
3. Senni K, Foucault-Bertaud A, Godeau G, et al. Magnesium and connective tissue. Mag Res. 2003;16:70-74.
4. Artaza JN, Norris KC. Vitamin D reduces the expression of collagen and key profibrotic factors by inducing an antifibrotic phenotype in mesenchymal mulitpotent cells. J Endocrinol. 2009;200:207-21.
5. Masuda I, Koike M, Nakashima S, et al. Apple procyanidins promote mitochondrial biogenesis and proteoglycan biosynthesis in chondrocytes. Sci Rep. 2018;8:7229.

6. Jean-Gilles D, Vaidyanathan VG, King R, et al. Inhibitory effects of polyphenol punicalagin on type-II collagen degradation in vitro and inflammation in vivo. Chem Biol Interact. 2013;205:90-92.

7. Lotz MK. Posttraumatic osteoarthritis: pathogenesis and pharmacological treatment options. Arth Res Ther. 2010;12:211.

8. Punzi L, Galozzi P, Luisetto R, et al. Post-traumatic arthritis: overview on pathogenic mechanisms and role of inflammation. RMD Open. 2016;2:e000279.

9. Zhuo Q, Yang W, Chen J, Wang Y. Metabolic syndrome meets osteoarthritis. Nat Rev Rheumatol. 2012;8:729-37.

10. Ford ES, Giles WH, Dietz WH. Prevalence of the metabolic syndrome among US adults. Findings from the Third National Health and Nutrition Examination Survey. J Am Med Assoc. 2002;287:356-59.

11. Goldenberg DL, Egan MS, Cohen AS. Inflammatory synovitis in degenerative joint disease. J Rheumatol. 1982;9:204-9.

12. Nakamura H et al. T-cell mediated inflammatory pathway in osteoarthritis. Osteoarthritis Cart. 1999;7:401-402.

13. Nishioka K. Autoimmune response in cartilage-derived peptides in a patient with osteoarthritis. Arth Res Ther 2003;6:6-7.

14. Kato T, Xiang Y, Nakamura H, Nishioka K. Neoantigens in osteoarthritic cartilage. Curr Opin Rheumatol. 2004;16:604-08.

15. Hopps E, Caimi G. Matrix metalloproteinases in metabolic syndrome. Eur J Int Med. 2012;23:99-104.

16. Derosa G, Maffioli P, D'Angelo A, et al. Effects of long chain omega-3 fatty acids on metalloproteinases and their inhibitors in combined dyslipidemia patients. Expert Opin Pharmacother. 2009;10:1239-47.

17. Li S, Niu G, Dong XN, Liu Z, Song C, Leng H. Vitamin D inhibits activities of metalloproteinase-9/-13 in articular cartilage in vivo and in vitro. J Nutr Sci Vitaminol. 2019;65:107-112.

18. Timms PM, Mannan N, Hitman GA, et al. Circulating MMP9, vitamin D and variation in the TIMP-1 response with VDR genotype: mechanisms for inflammatory damage in chronic disorders? Q J Med. 2002;95:787-96.

19. Kostov K, Halacheva L. Role of magnesium deficiency in promoting atherosclerosis, endothelial dysfunction, and arterial stiffening as risk factors for hypertension. Int J Mol Sci. 2018;19:1724.

20. Henrotin Y, Clutterbuck AL, Allaway D, et al. Biological actions of curcumin on articular chondrocytes. Osteoarthritis Cart. 2010;18:141-49.

21. Ahmed S, Wang N, Lalonde M, et al. Green tea polyphenol epigallocatechin-3-gallate (EGCG) differentially inhibits interleukin-1b-induced expression of matrix metalloproteinases-1 and -13 in human chondrocytes. J Pharmacol Exper Therapeutics. 2004;308:767-73.

22. Berenbaum F. Osteoarthritis as an inflammatory disease (osteoarthritis is not osteoarthrosis). Osteoarth Cart. 2013;21:16-21.

23. Schett G, Klyer A, Perricone C, et al. Diabetes is an independent predictor of severe osteoarthritis. Diabetes Care. 2013;36:403-409.

24. DeGroot J, Bank RA, Bijlsma JW, et al. Advanced glycation endproducts in the development of osteoarthritis. Arthritis Res Ther. 2004;6(Suppl 3):78.

25. Loeser RF, Yammani RR, Carlson CS, et al. Articular chondrocytes express the receptor for advanced glycation end products: potential role in osteoarthritis. Arth Rheum. 2005;52:2376-85.

26. Pearle AD, Warren RF, Rodeo SA. Basic science of articular cartilage and osteoarthritis. Clin Sports Med. 2005;24:1-12.

27. Pottie P, Presel N, Terlain B, et al. Obesity and osteoarthritis: more complex than predicted! Ann Rheum Dis. 2006;65:1403-05.

28. Tiku ML, Shah R, Allison GT. Evidence link chondrocyte lipid peroxidation to cartilage matrix protein degradation: possible role in cartilage aging and the pathogenesis of osteoarthritis. J Biol Chem. 2000;275:20069-76.

29. Tiku ML, Allison GT, Maik K, Karry SK. Malondialdehyde oxidation of cartilage collagen by chondrocytes. Osteoarthritis Cart. 2003;11:159-66.

30. Conaghan PG, Vanharanta H, Dieppe PS. Is progressive osteoarthritis an atheromatous vascular disease? Ann Rheum Dis 2005;64:1539-41.

31. Gkretsi V, Simopoulou T, Tsezou A. Lipid metabolism and osteoarthritis: lessons from atherosclerosis. Prog Lipid Res. 2011;50:133-40.

32. de Munter W, van der Kraon PM, van den Berg WB, van Lent PL. High systemic levels of low-density lipoprotein cholesterol: fuel to the flames of inflammatory osteoarthritis? Rheumatol. 2016;55:16-24.

33. Bonner WM, Jonsson H, Malanos C, Bryant M. Changes in the lipids of human cartilage with age. Arthritis Rheum. 1975;18:461-73.

34. Adkisson HD et al. Unique fatty acid composition of normal cartilage: discovery of high levels of n-9 eicosatrienoic acid and low levels of n-6 polyunsaturated fatty acids. FASEB J. 1991; 5(3):344-53.

35. Plumb MS, Aspden RM. High levels of fat and (n-6) fatty acids in cancellous bone in osteoarthritis. Lipids Health Dis. 2004,3:12.

36. Garfinkel RJ, Dilisio MF, Agrawal DK. Vitamin D and its effect on articular cartilage and osteoarthritis. Orthop J Sports Med. 2017;5(6):2325967117711376

37. Huang Z, Kraus VB. Does lipopolysaccharide-mediated inflammation have a role in OA? Nat Rev Rheumatol. 2016;12:123-29.

38. Chu SC, Yang SF, Lue KH, et al. Regulation of gelatinases expression by cytokines, endotoxin, and pharmacological agents in the human osteoarthritic knee. Connect Tissue Res. 2004;45:142-50.

39. Liu B, Zhang M, Zhao J, Zheng M, Yang H. Imbalance of M1/M2 macrophages is linked to severity level of knee osteoarthritis. Exp Therapeutic Med. 2018;16:5009-14.

40. Li Y, Luo W, Zhu S, Lei G. T cells in osteoarthritis: alterations and beyond. Front Immunol. 2017;8:356.

41. Reginster JY, Deroisy R, Rovati LC, et al. Long-term effects of glucosamine sulphate on osteoarthritis progression: a randomised, placebo-controlled clinical trial. Lancet. 2001;357:251-56.

42. Clegg DO, Reda DJ, Harris CL, et al. Glucosamine, chondroitin sulfate, and the two in combination for painful knee osteoarthritis. New Eng J Med. 2006; 354:795-808.

43. Bennett AN, Crossley KM, Brukner PD, Hinman RS. Predictors of symptomatic response to glucosamine in knee osteoarthritis: an exploratory study. Br J Sports Med 2007;41:415-419.

44. Pavelka K, Gatterova J, Olejarova M, et al. Glucosamine sulfate use and delay of progression of knee osteoarthritis: a 3-year, randomized, placebo-controlled, double-blind study. Arch Intern Med. 2002; 162:2113-23.

45. Srivastava KC, Mustafa T. Ginger (Zingiber officinale) in rheumatism and musculoskeletal disorders. Med Hypoth. 1992;39:342-48.

46. Li Y, Yue, Yang C. Unraveling the role of Mg++ in osteoarthritis. Life Sci. 2016;147:24-29.

47. Yao H, Xu JK, Zheng NY, et al. Intra-articular injection of magnesium chloride attenuates osteoarthritis progression in rats. Osteoarthritis Cart. 2019;27:1811-1821.

48. Zhang Y, Xu J, Qin L, Jiang Q. Magnesium and osteoarthritis: from a new perspective. Ann Joint. 2016;1:29

Chapter 16
Tendinosis: Diet-induced tendon rot

Chapter 14 about muscle degeneration began with an image of the various joint complex tissues. Below is the same Figure I used in Chapter 14. Notice again that muscles do not directly attach to bone. Instead, both sides of a muscle attach to a tendon, and it is the tendons that attach to bone.

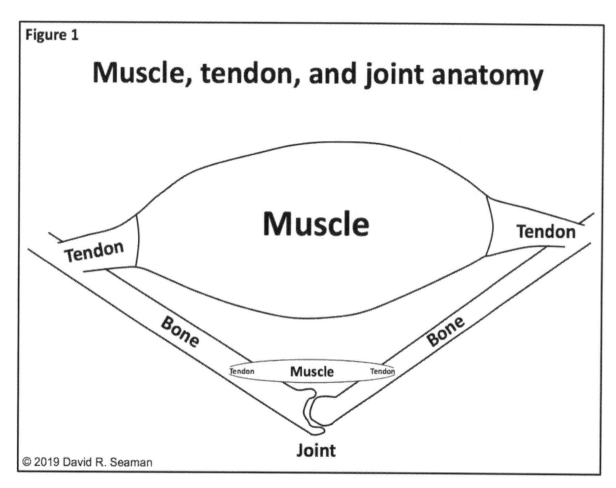

Figure 1

Muscle, tendon, and joint anatomy

© 2019 David R. Seaman

The term tendinopathy refers to both tendinitis and tendinosis. Most people have heard of tendinitis. In contrast, most people have not heard of tendinosis unless they are in the chiropractic, physical therapy, athletic trainer, or orthopedic professions. While the term tendinosis was first described in 1976 (1), it did not become a popular term until the mid to late 1990s. There are distinct differences between tendinitis and tendinosis.

Tendinitis vs tendinosis
Tendinitis is an acute inflammatory state in a tendon. It can develop from a single traumatic event or it can develop in a short time due to repeated excessive loads. Tendinitis typically resolves

between several days to 6 weeks, with a 99% likelihood of full recovery (2). Clinicians and research scientists maintain that tendinitis is a rare condition compared to tendinosis.

Tendinosis is a chronic condition caused by chronic overuse and it does not have a significant or obvious inflammatory presentation. This why tendinosis was initially and incorrectly viewed to be a non-inflammatory degenerative condition that was caused by wear-and-tear. Support for this misperception came from the observation that athletes like runners developed Achilles tendinosis and jumpers developed patella (knee cap) tendinosis. It is important to understand that these are typically healthy, young athletes that heal with rest and proper treatments. For these people, recovery time is about 6-10 weeks if tendinosis is identified early, but up to 6 months or longer if it is not identified until the chronic stage. The likelihood of full recovery is about 80% because tendons lack the abundant blood supply and recuperative abilities of muscle (2).

What complicates the tendinosis picture in the overall patient population is the fact that it also commonly develops in overweight non-exercisers who have the metabolic syndrome and type 2 diabetes. This means that tendinosis in the pro-inflammatory sedentary population is a different condition compared to the overuse tendinosis that occurs in healthy athletes. In short, researchers have begun to view tendinosis in the pro-inflammatory sedentary population as being similar to atherosclerotic heart disease (3), which means that it is a rotting condition of tendons just as atherosclerosis is a rotting condition of arteries. And this means that tendinosis in this population requires DeFlaming as their primary treatment.

Relevant tendon anatomy

In contrast to muscles and joint cartilage, tendons are not comprised mostly of water – the primary constituent of a tendon is collagen. As a quick review, as stated in Chapter 7, muscles are almost 80% water, joint cartilage is 70% water, and bones are 31% water. As described in Chapter 15, joint cartilage is comprised of collagen and proteoglycans, and the cells that make these substances are called chondrocytes (cartilage cells). The reason why cartilage contains so much water is because it must deal with compressive loads. In contrast, tendons never bear compressive loads, which is why they contain little water compared to muscles and joint cartilage.

As illustrated in Figure 1, shown earlier in this chapter, tendons lie between muscle and bone, and are pulled upon whenever a muscle contracts. This pulling load is called a tensile force or load. The greater the muscle contraction, the greater will be the tensile force applied to the tendons.

Although tendons contain water and proteoglycans, their primary component are collagen fibers that are needed in great abundance to deal with pulling/tensile forces (1). The primary cell type in tendons is called a tenocyte, which is a type of fibroblast (fibroblasts were discussed in Chapter 15). Tenocytes produce the collagen and proteoglycans that make up a tendon and keep it healthy. However, when the diet-induced pro-inflammatory state emerges, tenocytes become pro-inflammatory and drive tendon degeneration (rot).

Tendons contain a vascular supply, like most tissues, which means that immune cells, oxygen-containing red blood cells, and either a pro-inflammatory or anti-inflammatory state of body chemistry will move in and out of tendons when they are at rest and during activity. The last thing a tendon needs is for pro-inflammatory immune cells and body chemistry to enter the local tendon environment to augment the rotting pro-inflammatory state created locally in the tendon by pro-inflammatory tenocytes (4). The outcome is tendon degeneration and pain, and worse, possibly a rupture.

Tendon movement and chemistry production
In 2003, scientists published a study that looked at how simulated walking created blood flow in the Achilles tendon (5). While seated with their legs straight, the subjects in this study pressed into a pressure sensor plate at a level to mimic the tendon load created during normal walking. A microdialysis catheter was inserted through the Achilles tendon, which allowed for fluid collection in three states, those being during rest, simulated walking for 30 minutes, and recovery after simulated walking. The purpose was to measure blood flow during each of the three states when subjects were given a placebo or anti-inflammatory drugs such as ibuprofen and Celebrex.

Blood flow was increased during simulated walking and reduced back to normal during recovery in the subjects given the placebo, which is to be expected. This is an example of how movement is a chemical event, which was discussed previously in Chapter 7. One of the chemicals required for normal blood flow during motion is prostaglandin E2 (PGE2). If too little PGE2 is produced by tenocytes, blood flow will be reduced; however, if too much PGE2 is produced, the outcome will be inflammation and pain. Our bodies regulate this perfectly, so long as our diets are not pro-inflammatory.

When subjects in this simulated walking study were given Ibuprofen or Celebrex (anti-inflammatory drugs), there was measurable reduction in PGE2 production and a 35-43% reduction in blood flow below normal. This study demonstrated two important points. The first is that movement is definitely a chemical event. The second is that chronically taking anti-inflammatory drugs can rob tendons of their proper blood supply by suppressing tenocytes from producing a normal amount of PGE2. Regarding the latter, we now know that the chronic use of anti-inflammatory drugs can negatively affect tendon healing to create chronic non-healing tendinosis (6), which means that regular use of anti-inflammatory drugs can help to rot tendons.

This does not mean that anti-inflammatory drugs should never be used in the short term; but it does mean that no one should take them chronically as part of a lifestyle. Rather, the goal should be to create a DeFlamed state in the body that affords us the best chance to prevent diet-induced rotting of musculoskeletal tissues and to heal quickly after a painful injury.

Notice in Figure 2 that the muscle, tendon, and bone on the right side have been removed from what was shown in Figure 1. The normal tendon has lines in it, which represent normal collagen fiber orientation and next to it is a tendon with tendinosis that has lost its normal pattern of collagen fibers. The larger image contains the many pro-inflammatory factors that promote tendinosis in sedentary flamers, which are very similar to the pro-inflammatory factors that promote the other conditions described in previous chapters. Understanding these pro-inflammatory factors is quite relevant because about 30% of all pains that patients report to physicians involve painful tendons (7).

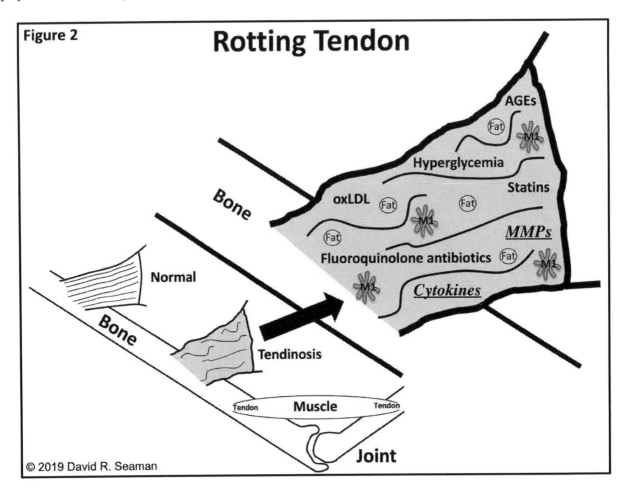

Notice also in Figure 2 that two classes of drugs can participate in promoting tendinosis. In the following sections, the various promoters of tendinosis will be discussed in more detail.

Drugs that weaken tendons

Toxic tendinopathy has been proposed as a term to characterize the tendon damage caused by certain medications (8). These medications include antibiotics, statins, and corticosteroids. Either avoiding these medications, or at least being very judicious with their use, can help to protect tendon health.

The flouroquinolone class of antibiotics have been linked to tendinopathy and tendon rupture. Carefully read the following quotation from an article that reviewed this topic (9):

"These adverse effects can occur within hours of commencing treatment and months after discontinuing the use of these drugs. In some cases, fluoroquinolone usage can lead to complete rupture of the tendon and substantial subsequent disability."

The many flouroquinolones to be aware of include ciprofloxacin (Cipro), levofloxacin (Levaquin), norfloxacin (Noroxin), gemifloxacin (Factive), and ofloxacin (Floxi)]. Research suggests that flouroquinolones damage tendons by stimulating the activity of matrix metalloproteinases (MMPs) (9), which are the connective tissue degrading enzymes discussed in previous chapters. These same enzymes caused tendinopathy, which is why they are included in Figure 2 in this chapter. Flouroquinolones also promote tendinopathy by inhibiting collagen synthesis (9).

Compared to the flouroquinolones, the relationship between statins and tendinopathy is less obvious. This is likely because a substantial number of patients taking statins are obese, insulin resistant, and hyperglycemic, which are risk factors for tendinopathy. Nonetheless, there does appear to be an increased risk of tendon pathology in patients taking statins compared to those that do not (10). This is potentially problematic, as multiple millions of Americans take statins every day for hypercholesterolemia and most of these same people are obese, insulin resistant, and hyperglycemic.

Corticosteroids, also called glucocorticoids, are a class of drugs that are almost identical to the hormone cortisol, which is produced by the adrenal glands. If too little is produced, body inflammation is not properly controlled. If too much is produced, it can be catabolic (degradative) to many tissues including tendons. When corticosteroids are taken long term, tendinopathy is a possible side-effect.

In summary, flouroquinolones appear to be the biggest concern for inducing tendon damage. This is even a problem for lean and fit individuals. If I had to take an antibiotic, I personally would never take a flouroquinolone, as other options are available.

Waist circumference and tendinosis

Consider a 45-year old male who is 50 pounds heavier than his leaner normal weight self when he was in college 25 years earlier. He decides to lose weight and jog to burn off extra calories. He starts jogging and within a month, he develops Achilles tendon pain, which is diagnosed as tendinopathy. It is very likely that he and his physician will think that the load created by jogging damaged the Achilles tendon...however, remember from earlier in this chapter that chronic overuse tendinopathy really only applies to healthy athletes. In the case of the overweight and obese population, tendinopathy typically exists in the sedentary population without symptoms. Here is a study that exemplifies this fact.

In order to understand how body fat mass promotes tendinopathy, scientists studied 298 people without Achilles tendinopathy symptoms (11). Diagnostic ultrasound was performed on 127 men and 171 women to identify the prevalence of tendinosis in people without tendon pain. In the male subjects, 13% had tendinosis, which translates into 17/127. All except one of the 17 men was 39 years or older and all but three of the men had a waist circumference greater than 33 inches. Thirteen of the 17 men were 45 years or older, reflecting that fact that as we get older and fatter, we are much more likely to develop tendon rot.

If we put this prevalence into a bigger picture, consider that there are 74 million men in America who are 40 years of age or older. At a 13% prevalence estimate, this suggests that almost 10 million men are walking around with rotting tendons and do not know it. Understand that this is an enormous number of people who will likely be mismanaged if they develop tendon pain.

Of the 171 women, only 5% had asymptomatic tendinopathy (meaning they showed no painful symptoms). However, all of the women with tendinopathy had a waistline of 27.5 inches or greater, as well as increased fat deposition in the hip region.

As described in Chapter 10, the pro-inflammatory cytokines released by obese adipose tissue cells leave the fat mass and enter circulation where they impact visceral and musculoskeletal tissues. In the context of this chapter, research suggests that tendons are flamed up and rotted by the pro-inflammatory cytokines released by obese adipose tissue, which leads to the development of tendinosis (12,13).

Insulin resistance and tendinopathy
Recall that insulin resistance was described in Chapter 12. Insulin resistance characterizes the pro-inflammatory metabolic syndrome and diabetes, which is a well-known promoter of tendinopathy as made exceptionally clear in the title of this article:

> Gaida JE, Alfredson L, Kiss ZS, et al. Dyslipidemia in Achilles tendinopathy is characteristic of insulin resistance. Med Sci Sports Exer. 2009;41:1194-97.

Notice the title of this article contains two key words, those being dyslipidemia and insulin resistance, which typically manifest simultaneously. The term dyslipidemia refers to elevated triglycerides, reduced HDL cholesterol, and elevated LDL cholesterol. Remember from Chapter 13 that what makes the cholesterol issue problematic is that both LDL and HDL become inflamed and oxidized. The term insulin resistance refers to a state of hyperglycemia and hyperinsulinemia, which is also associated with an elevated level of advanced glycation end products (AGEs).

As described in Chapter 13, the pro-inflammatory state of dyslipidemia and insulin resistance is what causes atherosclerosis. This same pro-inflammatory state causes tendinosis, which means that tendinosis is essentially atherosclerosis of tendons. This is why researchers have begun to view tendinosis as a type of cardiovascular disease (3). Recall from Chapter 15 that osteoarthritis is also being viewed biochemically as cardiovascular disease. In the remainder of this chapter, the dyslipidemia and insulin resistance issues will be discussed in the context of tendinosis.

oxLDL and tendinosis

In the human body, our connective tissues are continuously going through a remodeling process, which involves the degradation of old or damaged collagen and the subsequent synthesis of new collagen. This means that the collagen in my 60-year old tendons are not the same as when I was 40 or 20. In order for this remodeling process to be maintained, so that tendon integrity and health is maintained, tendon cells (tenocytes) need to regulate the synthesis and degradation of collagen. This can only happen if tenocytes are not pushed into a pro-inflammatory state by diet-induced dyslipidemia and insulin resistance.

When tenocytes are exposed to oxidized LDL cholesterol they behave in a pro-inflammatory fashion (14). Instead of maintaining a balance between collagen production and degradation, they begin to produce less collagen and overproduce MMPs that degrade the collagen, which leads to a net loss of collagen in tendons (15). In addition, cholesterol itself accumulates in tendons over time. This rotting process causes collagen fibers to weaken and become progressively less able to deal with normal loading over time, making them more prone to injury (16).

Hyperglycemia, AGEs, and tendinosis

As you obviously know by now, when we overeat sugar and flour, we create hyperglycemia, which becomes chronic over time. This also leads to the overproduction and accumulation of AGEs. In common language, this means that we "sugar-coat" our tendons, which leads to their degradation, stiffening, and weakening, and makes them prone to injury. The remainder of this section will describe this scenario in more detail.

As described earlier in the metabolic syndrome chapter, the over consumption of refined sugar and flour leads to hyperglycemia and eventually the metabolic syndrome and diabetes. Hyperglycemia itself promotes inflammation and also leads to an overproduction and accumulation of advanced glycation end products (AGEs) (17), which also promote inflammation.

As described in Chapters 6 and 12, the act of overeating refined sugar and flour will lead to a postprandial surge in blood glucose. Any cell exposed to this hyperglycemic state will release pro-inflammatory chemicals such as cytokines. This process occurs in tenocytes. When we are young, this hyperglycemic state is transient and related only to an overeating event and not likely to be especially damaging to any cell or tissue. However, as people age and develop the metabolic syndrome, they live in a 24-hour state of hyperglycemia. This will cause tenocytes and other cells to be perpetually bathed in excess glucose and lead to an overproduction of inflammatory chemicals, which prevents normal remodeling – collagen degradation is increased, while collagen synthesis is depressed (18). Hyperglycemia also leads to a reduced synthesis of proteoglycans (18,19).

Pentosidine is one of the better characterized advanced glycation end products (AGEs). Pentosidine levels are significantly elevated in patients with the metabolic syndrome compared to controls (17). Pentosidine levels gradually accumulate on tendon collagen over time, which reduces tendon elasticity (20), promotes tendon stiffness (21), and participates in the accelerated loss of range of motion that occurs in people who are pro-inflammaging. AGEs are known to suppress the activity of energy-producing mitochondria in tenocytes and reduce their connective tissue synthesizing capacity (21).

Vitamin D and matrix metalloproteinases
Chapter 11 discussed various functions of vitamin D. It turns out that adequate vitamin D is needed to prevent the overactivity of connective tissue-degrading matrix metalloproteinase enzymes (MMPs) (22). This means that without adequate vitamin D, there will be ineffective tendon remodeling, which will favor tendon degradation and tendinosis.

Pro-inflammatory immune cells in tendinosis
Similar to atherosclerosis, muscle rotting, and osteoarthritis, tendinosis is also characterized by a pro-inflammatory shift in immune cell activity (23), which was illustrated earlier in this chapter in Figure 2. This is essentially new evidence in the tendinosis literature and goes against "non-inflammatory mechanical injury dogma" that prevailed for many years. In 2018, researchers essentially stated that scientists and clinicians need to get over their cognitive dissonance and accept the fact that tendinosis is a pro-inflammatory condition (23).

From previous chapters, you might remember that endotoxin is pro-inflammatory and stimulates pro-inflammatory immune activity, which involves the release of cytokines and other inflammatory chemicals. While no studies have yet to look for localized endotoxin in people with tendinosis, future studies likely will. Despite this fact, we know that obesity and insulin resistance are related to rising levels of circulating endotoxin that will promote systemic and localized inflammation, which means that excess endotoxin is likely a promoter of tendinosis.

Important tendon anatomy changes with aging and chronic inflammation
As we age, tendon health declines, which is especially pronounced for people who are pro-inflammaging. The collagen fibers that make up the tendon undergo a process called "cross-linking," which is dramatically increased in people with the metabolic syndrome and diabetes. This helps to create the movement tightness that people feel as they age. There are likely multiple pro-inflammatory promoters of excessive cross-linking, but the most notable are advanced glycation end products (AGEs), which were discussed earlier in this chapter. Scientists call these AGE cross-links (20).

Summary
In a recent article published in 2019, the researchers stated that (21), "debilitating cases of tendon pain and degeneration affect the majority of diabetic individuals." In the previous chapter you saw that patients with diabetes are much more likely to have osteoarthritis. This means that the

dietary pursuit of diabetes (overeating refined sugar, flour, and oils) is also a pursuit of osteoarthritis and tendinosis. In the next chapter you will see that the same rotting process holds true for disc herniation.

The cross-linking and related reduced mobility that occurs with normal aging and worse, pro-inflammaging, is difficult to restore to levels comparable to younger individuals. This fact should be kept in mind whether one is aging normally or pro-inflammaging. If you are a flamer and want to exercise, you should choose your exercises carefully so that you gradually increase the load and intensity of exercise over time to avoid injuring tissues that have likely been flamed up for a long time.

References

1. Kaeding C, Best TM. Tendinosis: pathophysiology and nonoperative treatment. Sports Health. 2009;1:284-92.
2. Khan KM, Cook JL, Taunton JE, Bonar F. Overuse tendinosis, not tendinitis part 1: a new paradigm for a difficult clinical problem. Phys Sportsmed. 2000;28:38-48.
3. Gaida JE, Alfredson L, Kiss ZS, et al. Dyslipidemia in Achilles tendinopathy is characteristic of insulin resistance. Med Sci Sports Exer. 2009;41:1194-97.
4. Millar NL, Murrell GA, McInnes IB. Inflammatory mechanisms in tendinopathy – towards translation. Nature Reviews Rheumatology. 2017;13:110-122.
5. Langberg H, Boushel R, Skovgaard D, et al. Cyclo-oxygenase-2 mediated prostaglandin release regulates blood flow in connective tissue during mechanical loading in humans.J Physiol. 2003;551(Pt 2):683-9
6. Chan KM, Fu SC. Anti-inflammatory management for tendon injuries - friends or foes? Sports Med Arthrosc Rehabil Ther Technol. 2009;1:23.
7. Castro A, Skare TL, Nassif PA, et al. Tendinopathy and obesity. ABCD Arq Bras Cir Dig. 2016;29(Supl.1):107-10.
8. Bolon B. Mini-review: toxic tendinopathy. Toxicologic Path. 2017;45:834-37.
9. Lewis T, Cook J. Fluoroquinolones and tendinopathy: a guide for athletes and sports clinicians and a systematic review of the literature. J Athletic Training. 2014;49:422-27.
10. de Oliveira LP, Vieira CP, Da Re Guerrra F, et al. Statins induce biochemical changes in the Achilles tendon after chronic treatment. Toxicol. 2013;311:162-68.
11. Gaida JE, Alfredson L, Kiss ZS, et al. Assymptomatic Achilles tendon pathology is associated with a central fat distribution in men and a peripheral fat distribution in women: a cross sectional study of 298 individuals. BMC Musculoskelet Disord. 2010;11:41.
12. Gaida JE, Ashe MC, Bass SL, Cook JL. Is adiposity an under-recognized risk factor for tendinopathy? A systematic review. Arth Rheum. 2009;61:840-49.
13. Abate M. How obesity modifies tendons (implications for athletic activities). Muscles Ligaments Tendons J. 2014;4:298-302.
14. Scott A, Zwerver J, Grewal N, et al. Lipids, adiposity and tendinopathy: is there a mechanistic link? Critical review. Br J Sports Med. 2015;49:984-88.
15. Grewal N, Thornton GM, Behazad H, et al. Accumulation of oxidized LDL in the tendon tissues of C57BL/6 or apolipoprotein E knock-out mice that consume a high fat diet: potential impact on tendon health. PLoS One. 2014;9(12):e114214.

16. Steplewski A, Fertala J, Tomlinson R, et al. The impact of cholesterol deposits on the fibrillar architecture of the Achilles tendon in a rabbit model of hypercholesterolemia. J Orthopedic Surg Res. 2019;14:172.

17. Haddad M, Knani I, Bouzidi H, et al. Plasma levels of pentosidine, carboxymethyl-lysine, soluble receptor for advanced glycation end products, and metabolic syndrome: the Metformin effect. Dis Markers. 2016;2016:6248264.

18. Crownover J, Bielak K. Hyperglycemia and degenerative tendinopathy: a role for diet in tendon health. J Physical Rehab Med. 2015;1(3):015.

19. Burner T, Gohr C, Mitton-Fitzgerald E, Rosenthal AK. Hyperglycemia reduces proteoglycan levels in tendons. Connect Tissue Res. 2012;53:535-41.

20. Riley G. The pathogenesis of tendinopathy. A molecular perspective. Rheumatol. 2004;43:131-42. AGEs

21. Patel SH, Yue F, Saw SK, et al. Advanced glycation end products suppress mitochondrial function and proliferative capacity of Achilles tendon-derived fibroblasts. Sci Rep. 2019;9:Article:12614.

22. Dougherty KA, Dilisio MF, Agrawal DK. Vitamin D and the immunomodulation of rotator cuff injury. J Inflamm Res. 2016;9:123-131.

23. Mosca MJ, Rashid MS, Snelling SJ, Kirtley S, Carr AJ, Dakin SG. Trends in the theory that inflammation plays a causal role in tendinopathy: a systematic review and quantitative analysis of published reviews. BMJ Open Sport Exerc Med. 2018;4:e000332.

Chapter 17
Disc herniation: Diet-related disc rot

Disc degeneration and herniation are taught to doctors and therapists as being the outcome of trauma, not diet. The fact that a pro-inflammatory diet can promote disc degeneration and herniation is typically viewed as a fanciful notion. If you were to google search for diet-induced disc herniation, you would get the following:

Google

diet-induced disc herniation

Q All   Images   News   Videos   Shopping   More   Settings   Tools

About 954,000 results (0.76 seconds)

Scholarly articles for **diet-induced disc herniation**

The **diet-induced** proinflammatory state:: A cause of ... - Seaman - Cited by 87

Physical activity in daily life in patients with chronic low ... - Verbunt - Cited by 155

... and cytokine IL-1β in painful human intervertebral **discs** - Kepler - Cited by 71

Diet for disc herniation

Patients in pain, and particularly those with inflammatory **disc** conditions, i.e., discogenic and nerve root pain, should consume an anti-inflammatory **diet** that is relatively low in calories. The **food** focus should be omega-3 fish and eggs, lean meat and chicken, vegetables, fruit, and nuts (27).

The Chemistry of Discogenic and Disc Herniation Pain: Diet ...
https://www.anaboliclabs.com › NutraDisc_EducationalPieceFNL_2013_05

Search for: Diet for disc herniation

Notice that under scholarly articles, three are listed and mine is the first, which is specifically about the diet-induction of inflammation and pain. I also wrote *The Chemistry of Discogenic and Disc Herniation Pain: Diet and Nutritional Supplement Considerations* PDF document, which you can access if interested.

With the above in mind, there appears to be little evidence in the scientific literature that supports the fact that diet plays a role in disc degeneration or herniation. The reason for this is because diet is NOT typically viewed in the context of it being a key factor that determines a person's inflammatory status. Here is the proper perspective to maintain. A pro-inflammatory diet will lead to obesity, the metabolic syndrome, and diabetes, which then predisposes one to be more likely to develop all chronic diseases including disc herniation (1), but more importantly, these people are more likely to respond poorly to disc surgery and non-surgical conservative interventions (2,3), such as manipulation and rehabilitative exercise.

This chapter will outline how the chronic inflammatory state created by diet can promote disc degeneration and herniation. Before this relationship can be understood, you need to know some details about disc anatomy and the herniation process.

Painless disc degeneration and herniation

The title of this section was written properly. Disc degeneration and herniation can be completely painless, and most people are unaware of this fact that has been known for several decades.

In 1984, Dr. Sam Wiesel (Chairman of the Department of Orthopaedic Surgery at Georgetown University School of Medicine) and an Editor for a journal called Spine, made it very clear that disc herniations are very common in people with absolutely no symptoms at all (4). Indeed, based on CAT scans of the lumbar spine, 20% of subjects below 40 years of age had herniated discs. The number rose to 27% in those over 40. In 1991, a similar study on symptom-free subjects was performed using MRI imaging instead of CAT scans (5). In subjects under the age of 60, 22% had herniated discs, while 46% had degenerated discs. In those over 60, herniated discs were found in 46% of subjects, while 93% had degenerated discs.

Even if someone has disc herniation and pain, it does not mean that pain will continue so long as the disc remains herniated. In 1989, a case history was published about a patient who had a massive disc herniation in the low back. After receiving spinal manipulation, the pain was completely gone; however, a repeat CAT scan demonstrated that the disc herniation was unchanged.

So, what does all this mean? Very simply, the presence of disc herniation means that some people are completely pain-free, whereas others are writhing in pain. While all the questions to this paradox have not been answered, the best evidence suggests that for degenerated and herniated discs to be painful, there must be the presence of ongoing inflammation (6,7). Consider the fact that placing pressure on a nerve causes numbness and weakness but no pain. Inflammation is required for a nerve to become painful (7).

Disc and related anatomy

In this chapter you will learn about spinal anatomy so you can better appreciate the disc herniation process. The individual bones of the spine are called vertebra. The region of the neck is called the cervical spine; the mid back is called the thoracic spine, and the low back is called the lumbar spine. Since the low back is the most common area of herniation, the images created for this chapter are of the lumbar spine. Figure 1 is a side or lateral view of two lumbar vertebra and a disc. It is not an exact anatomical image, but it is accurate for the purposes of this discussion.

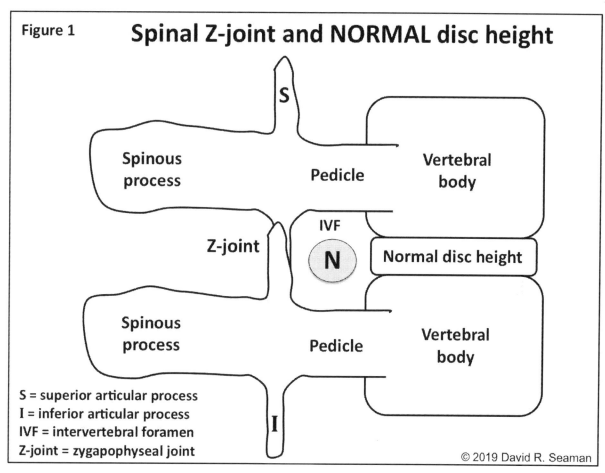

Figure 1 — **Spinal Z-joint and NORMAL disc height**

S = superior articular process
I = inferior articular process
IVF = intervertebral foramen
Z-joint = zygapophyseal joint

© 2019 David R. Seaman

The spinous process is the most posterior part of a vertebra. If you put your fingers into the middle of your low back you will be able to feel the tips of your spinous processes.

Spinal discs are located between the bodies of two vertebra, so they are called intervertebral discs. This relationship between vertebral bodies and the disc is referred to as the inter-body joint.

The Z-joint is the connection, or articulation, between the superior articular process of the vertebra below and the inferior articular process of the vertebra above. Both the Z-joints and the disc itself are common sources of spinal pain in the absence of disc herniation, which will be described more later in this chapter.

The intervertebral foramen (IVF) is where nerves exit from the spine. Notice that the top and bottom of the IVF is made up of a pedicle from each vertebra. The posterior area of the IVF is bordered by the Z-joint, while the disc and part of the superior and inferior vertebral bodies border the anterior area. You can see that the nerve (N) has plenty of room in the IVF, which means that it is not easily compressed or encroached upon. In fact, the IVF is normally 5-6 times the diameter of the spinal nerve that travels through it (8), which is why a loss in disc height is typically irrelevant as illustrated in Figure 2.

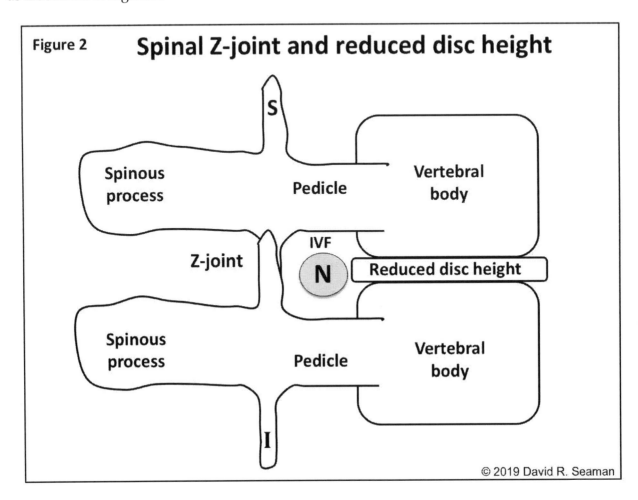

Notice that the disc is bulging into the IVF and yet there is still plenty of room for the nerve to exit the spine unencumbered. The likelihood that the nerve will be inflamed and painful is extremely unlikely; however, if there is pain, it will be coming from the Z-joint or the disc itself. The term discogenic pain is used to describe what is coming from the disc. As stated earlier, for the nerve to become painful it must become inflamed.

Figure 3 is an above-down view of the disc, Z-joint, IVF, nerve, and spinous process. The left sided image shows normal anatomy, while the image on the left illustrates pathological changes that can impact the nerve traveling through the IVF. Notice how the inferior (I) and superior (S) articular processes come together (articulate) to create the Z-joint, which is surrounded by the joint capsule and synovium (JC).

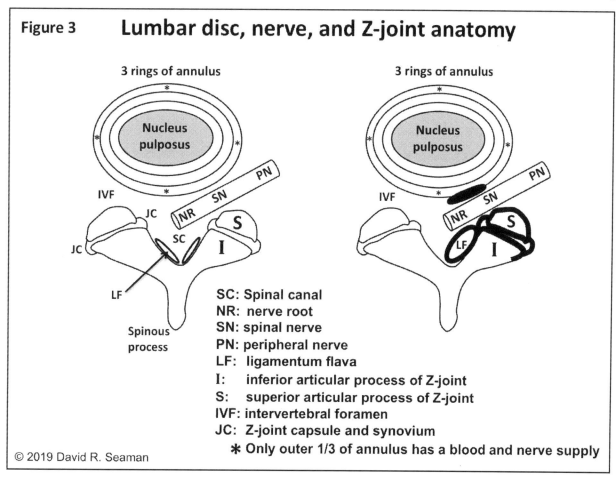

Figure 3 — Lumbar disc, nerve, and Z-joint anatomy

3 rings of annulus

Nucleus pulposus

IVF

PN

SN

JC

NR

SC

S

JC

I

LF

Spinous process

SC: Spinal canal
NR: nerve root
SN: spinal nerve
PN: peripheral nerve
LF: ligamentum flava
I: inferior articular process of Z-joint
S: superior articular process of Z-joint
IVF: intervertebral foramen
JC: Z-joint capsule and synovium
✱ Only outer 1/3 of annulus has a blood and nerve supply

© 2019 David R. Seaman

You can see the IVF between the Z-joint and disc. The spinal cord (not illustrated) is located in the spinal canal (SC). The back part of the spinal canal is bordered by a ligament called the ligamentum flava. Ligaments function to prevent excess movement.

The spinal cord descends from the brain and travels down the spinal canal. A total of 31 pairs of nerves branch off the spinal cord and leave the spine via the IVF. The term nerve root (NR) is used to describe the nerves that come off the spinal cord. Once the nerve roots reach the IVF, they are referred to as spinal nerves (SN). After a spinal nerve leaves the IVF, it is now called a peripheral nerve (PN). Later in this chapter you will see why it is important to understand the differences between the NR, SN, and PN.

Notice now that the disc is made up of two distinct component parts. In the middle is the nucleus pulposus, which is called the nucleus for short. The nucleus is mostly made of proteoglycans, which is surrounded by the annulus fibrosus, which is called the annulus for short. The annulus is made up of mostly collagen fibers.

The annulus is typically illustrated as being divided into thirds, which I am calling 3 rings. Only the outer third of the annulus has a blood and nerve supply, which means that only the outer third of the annulus can become painful. This topic will be discussed later in this chapter.

The image on the right illustrates anatomy changes that can narrow the IVF and make it more difficult for the nerve to move. Most people do not realize that nerves move, but they do. When you bend forward, backwards, sideways, and rotate, the nerves leaving the spine will slightly move and we want this movement to be free, unencumbered, and not associated with inflammation. Several degenerative changes can occur that can narrow the IVF.

On the right side you can see that an area of the disc is bolded, illustrating a narrowing effect on the IVF. The articular process can hypertrophy (get bigger) and add to the narrowing effect. The Z-joint capsule can become inflamed and hypertrophied. The ligamentum flava also commonly hypertrophies and adds to narrowing of the spinal canal. Advanced glycation end-products, which were described in previous chapters, are increased in the hypertrophied ligamentum flava of patients with diabetes, which is one of the reasons why people with type 2 diabetes are more likely to develop spinal canal narrowing (stenosis) compared to non-diabetics (9). It is important to understand that all of these changes can occur and still many people feel little to no pain at all!

The key and determining factor in pain expression, no matter where the pain is, has to do with the presence or absence of inflammation. For some people the various encroachment factors and inflammation are so severe that surgery is the only option. However, many people have thoroughly DeFlamed themselves and avoided surgery. While we cannot correct the anatomical changes that may develop as we age, we can certainly control our inflammatory state.

I personally have most of the anatomical changes I just discussed and have either no pain or minor/mild pain, and am able to play golf, surf, do yard work, and exercise. That could change as I age, but for now at age 60 I am doing pretty good and cannot imagine how bad I would feel if I flamed up my diet.

Disc anatomy that you need to know about
It turns out that the entire disc herniation process is an inflammatory event (6). This can be easily understood when you understand more details about disc anatomy. Figure 4 illustrates the anatomy of the disc. In the top right-hand corner of the figure, notice it looks kind of like a sandwich, with the two vertebral bodies as pieces of bread and the disc as the meat. By cutting the sandwich in half, you would be able to see what the middle looks like, and that is what you see in Figure 4.

The title of Figure 4 is "Spinal disc complex anatomy." The reason for this title is that the disc is intimately associated with the vertebral endplates and bodies. Notice how the annulus is imbedded in the endplate and vertebral body. It turns out that the endplates are the key structure of the disc complex when it comes to understanding disc biology and herniation.

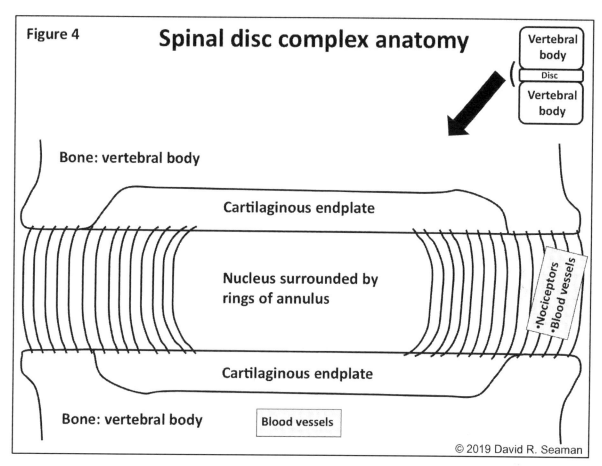

Figure 4

Spinal disc complex anatomy

Vertebral body
Disc
Vertebral body

Bone: vertebral body

Cartilaginous endplate

Nucleus surrounded by rings of annulus

•Nociceptors
•Blood vessels

Cartilaginous endplate

Bone: vertebral body

Blood vessels

© 2019 David R. Seaman

The cartilaginous endplate is similar to the articular or joint cartilage found in joints, as described in Chapter 15. The endplate also has no blood supply or nerve supply (nociceptors), which makes it the perfect interface between the boney vertebral body and the nucleus. The vertebral body contains a blood supply, while the nucleus contains no blood or nerve supply (nociceptors). The inner 2/3s of the annulus that surrounds the nucleus also has no blood or nerve supply. Nutrients get to the endplate, inner annulus, and nucleus through a body movement-driven diffusion process from blood vessels in the vertebral body and outer annulus.

The nucleus consists of up to 85% water, which means that it is the perfect structure for dealing with compressive forces - remember that water is essentially incompressible. Recall from the joint chapter that water is imbibed by proteoglycans made by chondrocytes. In the disc nucleus, proteoglycans are produced by fibroblasts.

A healthy nucleus and associated annulus are so strong that severe compressive forces will damage the vertebral body and endplate, but not the nucleus or annulus (10). With this in mind, it has been known for a long time that the first unequivocal event that begins the disc herniation process is damage to the endplate and subsequent inflammatory degradation of the nucleus (10). The moment the end plate is damaged enough to compromise the nucleus, the annulus is forced to deal with unaccustomed compressive forces that would otherwise be dealt with by the nucleus (11).

Endplate damage and disc herniation

Damage to the endplate can cause a little blood from the vertebral body to enter the endplate that otherwise never has blood in it, which can then get into the nucleus. Once a little blood gets into the nucleus, either the immune cells in the blood or the fibroblasts in the nucleus are activated to begin producing MMPs. Recall that MMPs stands for matrix metalloproteinases, which is a family of enzymes that degrade proteoglycans and collagen. Figure 5 illustrates what happens when MMPs degrade the nucleus and annulus.

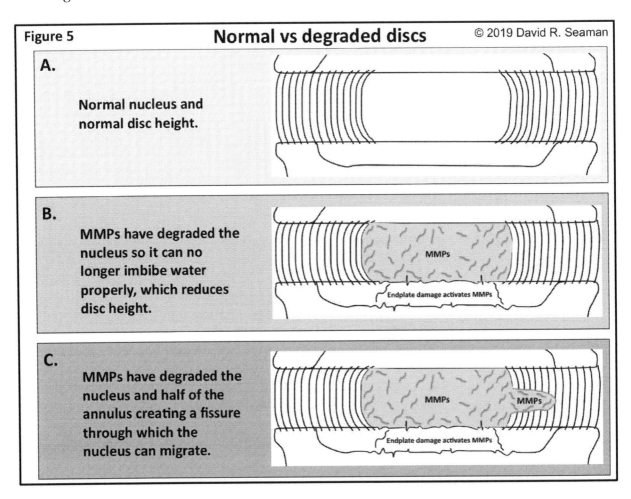

Figure 5 — Normal vs degraded discs — © 2019 David R. Seaman

A. Normal nucleus and normal disc height.

B. MMPs have degraded the nucleus so it can no longer imbibe water properly, which reduces disc height. (MMPs; Endplate damage activates MMPs)

C. MMPs have degraded the nucleus and half of the annulus creating a fissure through which the nucleus can migrate. (MMPs; MMPs; Endplate damage activates MMPs)

Perhaps the most important point to understand about Figure 5 is that endplate damage and disc degradation can occur without any symptoms at all. The reason is that neither the endplate, nucleus, or inner annulus have a nerve supply, so no pain experience can occur despite the damage that has taken place.

Figure 5A illustrates a normal disc. In contrast, Figure 5B illustrates a disc that has lost its height compared to the normal disc. The reason is because the MMPs have digested the proteoglycans in a fashion that no longer allows them to properly imbibe water. If the MMPs remain active, they will continue to degrade the annulus, as illustrated in Figure 5C. This migration pattern is called a radial fissure.

It is very important to understand that a normal nucleus is a cohesive structure that has no flowing capacity at all because it is not fluid-like. In contrast, a degraded nucleus has been rendered fluid-like and can migrate into radial fissures. Believe it or not, the best way to conceptualize this is with Jell-O, which is much less strong and cohesive than the nucleus but serves as a good example. Jell-O retains its shape after it is made. It can even retain its shape when it is jiggled and can also support weight to a certain degree, very much like the nucleus.

Jell-O is made from collagen that has been extracted from animal muscles, bones, and skin, which is then called gelatin. Jell-O can be made with any freshly cut fruit except for pineapples and the reason is because freshly cut pineapples contain an enzyme called bromelain, which digests gelatin. If fresh pineapples are used, the outcome is soupy Jell-O that is fluid-like compared to the cohesive Jell-O that most people have seen. In other words, the bromelain from pineapples is to Jell-O as MMPs are to the proteoglycans of the nucleus and collagen of the annulus.

MMPs are regulated by inhibitors called tissue inhibitors of metalloproteinases (TIMPs), which stop MMPs from digesting proteoglycans and collagen. At any point after MMPs are activated, they can be turned off by TIMPs. If this happens early enough in the process, MMPs will not digest the annulus. If the MMPs are turned off, the degradation will stop and viable fibroblasts in the nucleus will hopefully pump out collagen to make the nucleus fibrous no longer fluid-like, which is what happens during the normal aging process (12).

In Figure 5C, you can see that the MMPs have stopped digesting collagen about halfway into the annulus. MMPs can be inhibited at this point or earlier, or they can remain free to digest collagen all the way into the outer third of the annulus. If the latter happens, the next step is herniation, which will be explained shortly. But for now, it is important to know that the scenario I just outlined was described by scientists as an inflammatory degradation process at least as early as 1991 (6), which means it has been known for many years. We now know that the degrading disc contains MMPs, free radicals, prostaglandins, cytokines, and an acidic pH (13-15), and likely other inflammatory chemicals.

Notice in Figure 6 that nociceptors and blood vessels populate the outer third of the annulus. Nociceptors are specialized nerve cells that sense inflammation and generate the experience of pain. If the inflammatory degradation of the nucleus and annulus extends to the outer third of the annulus, nociceptors can be activated to cause pain, which is referred to as discogenic pain (see Figure 6). For some the pain is barely noticeable, while for others the pain can be debilitating.

I should mention that it is generally difficult to conceptualize why some people experience no pain or severe debilitating pain if they have the same inflammatory degradation pattern extending into the heavily innervated (lots of nociceptors) outer third of the annulus. In short, no one knows why this is the case. The most likely reason has to do with an individual's unique biochemistry and physiology, which is based on our genetic makeup. Some people are genetically more likely to express inflammation and pain more than others (16-19).

As stated above, once the migrating inflammatory exudate of the nucleus reaches the outer third of the annulus and pain manifests, it is called discogenic pain. This means that the genesis of the pain is from the disc. It is also called primary disc pain to distinguish it from the pain of disc herniation.

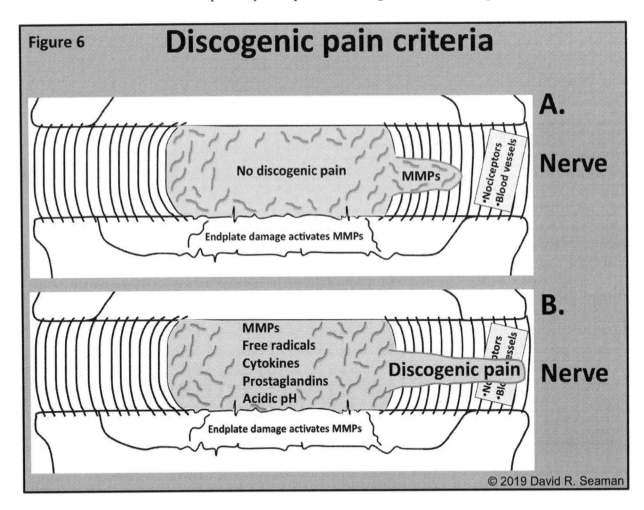

In the late 1980s, the disc herniation sequence was outlined and codified based on what is called a discogram. Patients would have dye injected into the suspected discs and then be CAT scanned to identify the status of a painful disc. Discograms are rarely if ever performed anymore, as MRI scans are able to identify the progression of herniation very easily.

Figure 7 illustrates the discogram herniation classification system, which goes from Grade 0 to Grade 5. In Grade 0, the nucleus can be digested to varying degrees; but either way, the annulus is not compromised by the degradative process described earlier. However, when the nucleus undergoes the degradation process it is no longer able to handle the compressive loads that it could when it was normal. When this happens, the annulus begins to take a compressive burden it was not built to handle (11). This can eventually cause collagen layers to delaminate (*) as illustrated in Grades 0-2 in Figure 7. The degree to which this happens can vary substantially among patients.

Notice that in Grade 1, the nucleus has migrated into the inner third of the annulus, which means that MMPs had to be at work to degrade the annulus. Notice also that the delamination of the annulus is worse in Grade 1, compared to Grade 0.

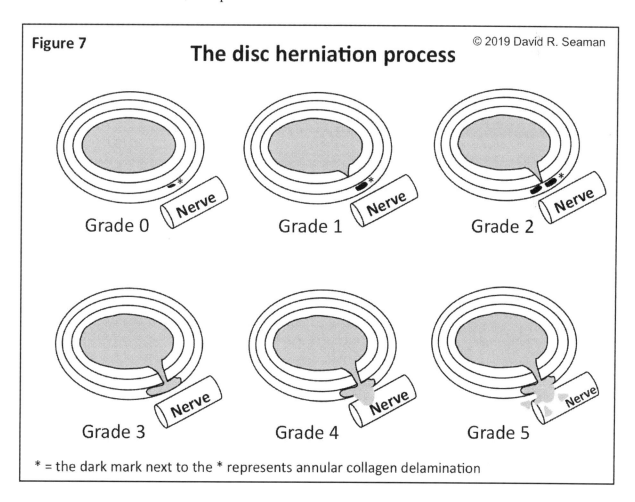

Figure 7 © 2019 David R. Seaman

The disc herniation process

Grade 0　　Nerve

Grade 1　　Nerve

Grade 2　　Nerve

Grade 3　　Nerve

Grade 4　　Nerve

Grade 5　　Nerve

* = the dark mark next to the * represents annular collagen delamination

If the degradation process continues, the nucleus can migrate into the middle third of the annulus, which is referred to as Grade 2. Annular delamination (*) has also progressed compared to Grades 0 and 1. At this point, if a patient is in pain, the source of the pain is likely to be coming from the Z-joints and not the disc itself or the nearby nerve traveling through the IVF, as neither has been compromised by the inflammatory exudate.

When a patient transitions from Grade 2 to Grade 3, severe pain may manifest as a load of prostaglandins and cytokines are delivered to the nociceptor-rich outer annulus that has been previously delaminated (*). A patient with a Grade 3 discogram is said to have discogenic pain. It is possible that this patient may now have two sources of pain, one being the Z-joint and the other being the disc.

Notice also in Grade 3 that the nucleus-derived inflammatory exudate can travel around the annulus, which means it can stimulate more nociceptors to enhance the level of pain. If the nucleus herniates through the outer annulus, the nerve root and spinal nerve will be exposed to the inflammatory exudate, which will be classified as either Grade 4 or Grade 5.

In a Grade 4 disc, the nuclear exudate remains intact, compared to a Grade 5 herniation wherein fragments of the nucleus are noticeable. The degree of pain between a Grade 4 and 5 may be negligible or dramatic. It is even possible for a Grade 4 to be more painful than a Grade 5. Additionally, when pain is present in a Grade 4 or 5, it is likely to have three sources of nociception, those being the Z-joint, the outer annulus (discogenic pain), and the nerve root and/or spinal nerve. When there is nerve root pain, it is called radicular pain. Radix is latin for root, and thus the term radicular mean that pain is coming from the root.

Discogenic pain versus radicular pain

Low back pain is one of the most common conditions from which people suffer. The source of the pain varies, but there are four primary sources. Just about 5% of all back pain involves a herniated disc that stimulates the nerve root; however, 40% of back pain is discogenic (20,21). In other words, the discogenic pain process I described above outlines the most common mechanism of back pain generation.

Another 20% of pain comes from the sacroiliac joint. Depending on age, between 15-40% comes from Z-joints (20,21). Older people tend to have more Z-joint pain than younger individuals.

From a mechanistic perspective, discogenic, sacroiliac, and Z-joint pains are identical. Each is caused by the stimulation of nociceptors in the respective tissues by inflammatory chemicals. Radicular pain is a very different based on the anatomy of nerves.

In Figure 8, notice the nociceptor beginning in the outer annulus being stimulated by the inflammatory exudate from the herniated nucleus. This is how inflammation stimulates nociceptors in any tissue that hurts, such as joints, muscles, tendons, bone, and visceral tissues, the most common being gut pain. Once the nociceptor beginning is stimulated by inflammation, the nociceptor axon transmits the "inflammation" message to the nociceptor terminal in the spinal cord, which then activates another nerve cell that conducts the "inflammation" message to the brain where it is experienced as pain.

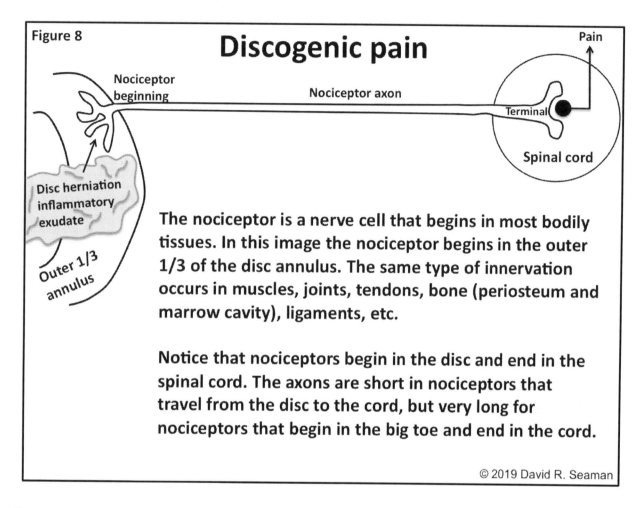

Figure 8

Discogenic pain

Nociceptor beginning

Nociceptor axon

Pain

Terminal

Spinal cord

Disc herniation inflammatory exudate

Outer 1/3 annulus

The nociceptor is a nerve cell that begins in most bodily tissues. In this image the nociceptor begins in the outer 1/3 of the disc annulus. The same type of innervation occurs in muscles, joints, tendons, bone (periosteum and marrow cavity), ligaments, etc.

Notice that nociceptors begin in the disc and end in the spinal cord. The axons are short in nociceptors that travel from the disc to the cord, but very long for nociceptors that begin in the big toe and end in the cord.

© 2019 David R. Seaman

The nature of discogenic pain is very similar to pain from joints, tendons, muscles, and bone. It is typically a deep achy feeling that is diffuse, which means spread out and difficult to specifically localize. Radicular or nerve pain is very different. It is deep, sharp, searing, especially intense, and noticeably different from pain originating in discs, muscles, joints, tendons, or bone. Any movement or position that puts tension on the nerve can cause brutal pain, such as movement of the arm or leg. Bearing down, as during a bowel movement, can also activate the pain experience.

To understand the nature of radicular pain, which is sometimes incorrectly called sciatica or sciatic pain, a bit of easy-to-understand neuroanatomy information is required. Figure 9 is a build upon Figure 8.

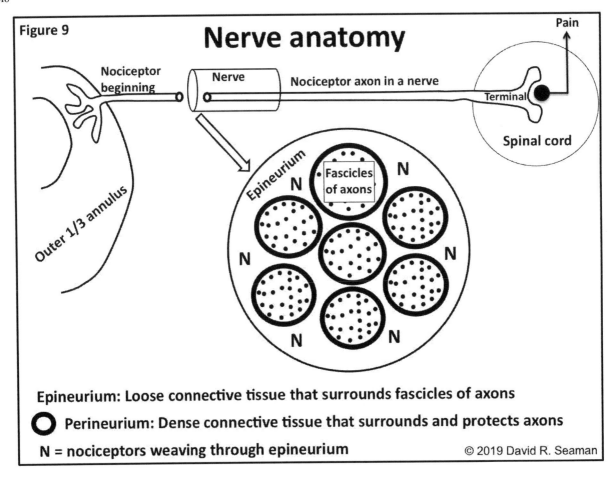

Figure 9

Nerve anatomy

Pain

Nociceptor beginning

Nerve

Nociceptor axon in a nerve

Terminal

Spinal cord

Outer 1/3 annulus

Epineurium

Fascicles of axons

N

Epineurium: Loose connective tissue that surrounds fascicles of axons

Perineurium: Dense connective tissue that surrounds and protects axons

N = nociceptors weaving through epineurium

© 2019 David R. Seaman

Recall that nociceptors are nerve cells that sense inflammation. A nociceptor has a beginning that senses the inflammation, an axon that transmits the "inflammation" message to the spinal cord, and a nociceptor terminal that stimulates a spinal cord nerve cell that takes information to the brain where pain is experienced. Figures 8, 9, and 10 illustrate just one nociceptor innervating the disc; however, in our bodies, there can be many hundreds, if not more, nociceptors that innervate our various individual body tissues.

Notice that the nerve and the nociceptor traveling in the nerve have been cut so you can see inside the nerve to get a better appreciation for its anatomy. A nerve is a unique anatomical structure. Notice that there are fascicles, or bundles, of axons. The majority of axons in any nerve will be nociceptor axons, which has been known for many years (23,24). The fascicles of axons are protected by a dense ring of connective tissue made of collagen called perineurium, which are surrounded by a loose type of connective tissue called epineurium that is also made of collagen.

It turns out that the connective tissue that makes up the epineurium and perineurium is similar to the connective tissue in muscles, tendons, joints, and outer annulus of the disc. Another similarity is that the epineurium is also innervated with nociceptors. This means that stimulation of nociceptors within the epineurium can create pain similar to that from other musculoskeletal tissues. The big difference in pain experience occurs when axons are exposed to inflammation. This leads to the excruciating deep, sharp, and searing nerve pain mentioned earlier.

I have personally experienced this nerve or radicular pain myself. One of the joint capsules in my lumbar spine developed a synovial cyst, which fortunately resorbed on its own. However, while it was active, the pain was intense. My situation was atypical. The only time I had any pain was when I did anything to traction the nerves in my right leg. If I was standing up and flexed my chin to my chest, the pain exploded down my leg and caused a deep boring pain in my right ankle...I never felt anything like this before.

The interesting thing for me was that I had essentially no pain at all when I did not traction the nerves in my leg. I cannot say for sure, but it is likely that because I was otherwise not living a pro-inflammatory lifestyle, my body chemistry was not especially inflamed and therefore, not perpetually feeding more inflammation to the inflamed nerve root in my fifth lumbar spine region.

The pain eventually resolved on its own and I have been free of the symptoms for almost 15 years. Figure 10 illustrates why disc herniation can be so painful.

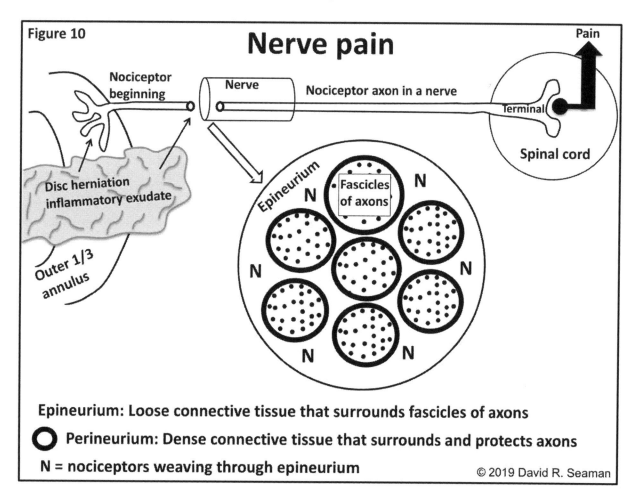

Figure 10

Nerve pain

Nociceptor beginning

Nerve

Nociceptor axon in a nerve

Pain

Terminal

Spinal cord

Disc herniation inflammatory exudate

Outer 1/3 annulus

Epineurium

Fascicles of axons

N

N

N

N

N

N

N

Epineurium: Loose connective tissue that surrounds fascicles of axons

○ **Perineurium: Dense connective tissue that surrounds and protects axons**

N = nociceptors weaving through epineurium

© 2019 David R. Seaman

Before a disc herniates, there would only be discogenic pain, caused by the inflammatory exudate stimulating only nociceptors in the outer annulus. After the nucleus and inflammatory exudate moves out of the disc, it can stimulate the nerve root and/or spinal nerve. When this happens, you get an additional double dose of nociceptor stimulation on top of the discogenic pain. First, the inflammatory chemicals seep into the epineurium to stimulate the nociceptors that populate the epineurium. When this happens, it can feel like the discogenic pain doubles. Second, the inflammatory chemicals seep deeper into the fascicles and directly activate the axons of potentially hundreds of nociceptors...this is what causes the excruciating pain that drives some people to opioid medications and surgery.

To summarize, the inflammatory exudate associated with disc herniation will stimulate nociceptor beginnings in both the outer annulus and epineurium, which is bad enough and something you would not wish on an enemy. But it gets many times worse when hundreds of nociceptor axons are activated by the inflammatory exudate.

It took about a month or two before my nerve root pain crisis was completely gone. The synovial cyst resorbed and I was fine. Fortunately, herniated disc material also resorbs.

Resorption of herniated material
Resorb and resorption refer to the gradual breakdown of a tissue or structure into component materials and its dispersal into circulation. Many studies have confirmed that herniated disc material can be resorbed (24-27). In one case study a patient was followed over 3 years. Notice the title of this article:

> Reyentovich A, Abdu WA. Multiple, sequential, and spontaneously resolving lumbar intervertebral disc herniations: a case report. Spine. 2002;27:549-53.

The patient in this case report suffered through three large lumbar disc herniations during a three-year period. Each one resorbed on its own, which was followed by a pain-free period of time that was interrupted by another herniation.

The time frame is typically within 2 months to a year for a herniated disc to resorb, so the term "spontaneous resorption" should not be viewed as an instantaneous event. In my experience, the resorption process appears to be much more successful if one is DeFlamed or begins to aggressively DeFlame themselves during the herniation and resorbing process. In fact, DeFlaming has saved many people from having surgery due to a herniated disc.

How physical trauma can masquerade as the key cause of disc herniation
When people conceptualize physical trauma, we undoubtedly will think of some injurious event that causes immediate pain. Virtually no one thinks physical trauma can be pain-free. But that is the nature of the painless endplate damage that sets in motion the painless inflammatory

degradation that heal and never cause symptoms, or it can ultimately lead to severe discogenic and herniation pain.

Let's consider a generic 45-year old male that has lived a pro-inflammatory lifestyle, and has a Grade 2 disc, but with minimal to no pain. This means he has no idea he is just a single disc grade away from potentially severe discogenic back pain.

He tries to stay active like many middle-age men who are stressed out, overweight, not sleeping well, and overeating refined food calories. Despite these poor lifestyle choices, he thinks he is basically doing okay because he doesn't have much body pain and basically no back pain at all. However, like many 45-year old men, he has the metabolic syndrome and is taking an anti-hypertensive drug, a statin for high cholesterol, and metformin for high blood sugar.

Then one day he plays golf and coincidently moves from a Grade 2 disc into a painful Grade 3 disc, which would have happened anyway; HOWEVER, the timing of pain expression was associated with physical activity, which makes him think that the trauma from playing golf was the cause. Within a week, his disc becomes a Grade 4 disc and he is now writhing in pain with both nociceptive and ectopic nociceptive pain.

The only cause-effect relationship he has in his brain is that playing golf caused his brutal pain, which could have coincidentally happened while watching TV, playing softball, sitting at his desk, or doing yard work. He goes to see a doctor and has an MRI done and is shown the herniated disc, so he naturally thinks that physical activity damaged the disc and caused a herniation. This incorrect belief is quite problematic because it causes the mind to fear future physical activity.

Accordingly, the doctor should correct his incorrect perception about physical activity and disc herniation – he should be told very clearly by his doctor that normal physical activities and labor do not cause discs to herniate. For perspective, he should have also been told that pro-inflammatory people with metabolic syndrome or diabetes are basically rotting and are more likely to herniate discs and/or develop osteoarthritis, tendinosis, osteoporosis, heart disease, and cancer, compared to normal anti-inflammatory people. The images in this book and chapter are designed to help properly conceptualize these factual relationships.

Treating herniated discs
The most important thing to know is that herniated discs naturally resorb as described in the *Resorption of herniated material* section of this chapter. The primary goal of a patient should be to avoid surgery if they can, which is the case for most people. Pain cannot be used as an indicator for surgery, which instead should be based on a progressive loss of neurologic integrity. This means the development and worsening of muscle weakness and a loss of muscle reflexes. In the case of lumbar disc herniation, a progressive loss of bladder and bowel control also indicates a loss of neurologic integrity. If these neurologic changes are absent, then there is no need for surgery in

most cases. In the absence of progressing neurologic deficits, pain control is the most important issue of care for all people with painful herniated discs and this is because some people still opt for surgery because of severe pain.

As long as pain can be reduced to a tolerable level, the natural resorption process will take place without the need for surgery. Opioid drugs for pain control should be the last medication of choice due to their addictive nature, especially for those with depression and/or anxiety. Consider the fact that 80% of all opioid addicts begin with a prescription from a medical doctor to treat a painful condition.

If I had a painful herniated disc and needed medication, I would opt for the short-term use of corticosteroids and NSAIDs. I would also utilize all conservative treatments possible, which are offered by most chiropractors and physical therapists who specialize in spine care.

Not surprisingly, I would also strictly adhere to The DeFlame Diet and endeavor to get all of my inflammatory markers into the normal range as soon as possible. The supplements discussed in Chapter 9 can be helpful in this endeavor.

In the final section of this chapter, I will outline the dietary factors that help to promote disc herniation. Not surprisingly, they mirror the dietary factors that cause heart disease, muscle rotting, osteoarthritis, and tendinosis.

Diet-induced inflammation and disc herniation

As outlined earlier in this chapter, endplate damage sets in motion the disc herniation process. This can happen with a single traumatic event or due to repetitive activities performed over time. In no way does poor nutrition initiate the process, but it does influence the nucleus degradation and herniation process. This is best appreciated when we use the metabolic syndrome and type 2 diabetes as examples of diet-induced pro-inflammatory states that places people at greater risk for disc herniation compared to normal subjects (28-31). One of the reasons for this is that chronic hyperglycemic states like metabolic syndrome and diabetes are associated with greater activity of matrix metalloproteinases (MMPs) (32,33), which, as described earlier in this chapter, participate in the disc herniation process.

As I described previously in Chapter 15, to normalize MMP activity, my perception is that we should get our metabolic syndrome markers into the normal range, and additionally consider taking the key supplements to help reduce inflammation and regulate MMP activity, those being omega-3 fatty acids, vitamin D, magnesium, and polyphenols (34-39).

Research has demonstrated that oxidized LDL (ox-LDL) cholesterol can stimulate MMPs to degrade the nucleus and promote disc herniation (40). Accordingly, people with elevated triglycerides and ox-LDL cholesterol are more likely to develop disc herniation (41).

Advanced glycation end products (AGEs) appear to have the ability to enter the nucleus and participate in the initiating of disc herniation by stimulating MMPs (42). AGE levels can also accumulate in spinal nerves and participate in pain induction after disc herniation (43).

As described in Chapter 10 about obesity, there is an increased release of leptin by obese fat cells. It turns out that leptin may also stimulate MMPs to degrade the nucleus and cause herniation (44).

Clearly, the pro-inflammatory state induced by obesity, the metabolic syndrome, and diabetes is a promoter of disc herniation. So, in addition to various treatment options available to patients, they should also become thoroughly DeFlamed.

References

1. Seaman DR. Body mass index and musculoskeletal pain: is there a connection? Chiropractic Man Ther. 2013;21:15.
2. Rihn JA, Kurd M, Hilibrand AS, et al. The influence of obesity on the outcome of treatment of lumbar disc herniation. Analysis of the Spine Patient Outcomes Research Trial (SPORT). J Bone Joint Surg Am. 2013;95:1-8.
3. Glassman SD, Alegre G, Carreon L, Dimar JR, Johnson JR. Perioperative complications of lumbar instrumentation and fusion in patients with diabetes mellitus. Spine J. 2003;3:496-501.
4. Wiesel SW, Tsourmas N, Feffer HL, Citrin CM, Patronas N. A study of computer-assisted tomography. I. The incidence of positive CAT scans in an asymptomatic group of patients. Spine. 1984;9:549-51.
5. Boden SD, Davis DO, Dina TS, Patronas NJ, Wiesel SW. Abnormal magnetic-resonance scans of the lumbar spine in asymptomatic subjects. A prospective investigation. J Bone Joint Surg Am. 1990;72:403-8.
6. Bogduk N, Twomey LT. Clinical anatomy of the lumbar spine. 2nd ed. New York: Churchill Livingstone; 1991: p.168-170.
7. Bogduk N. On the definitions and physiology of back pain, referred pain, and radicular pain. Pain. 2009;147:17-19.
8. Boden SD, Wiesel SW, Laws ER, Rothman RH. The aging spine: essentials of pathophysiology, diagnosis, and treatment. Philadelphia: Saunders; 1991: p.18.
9. Maruf MH, Suzuki A, Hayashi K, et al. Increased advanced glycation end products in hypertrophied ligamentum flavum of diabetes mellitus patients. Spine J. 2019;19:1739-45.
10. Adams M, Bogduk N, Burton K, Dolan P. The biomechanics of back pain. New York: Churchill Livingstone; 2002: p.133, 147
11. Adams MA, Roughley PJ. What is intervertebral disc degeneration, and what causes it? Spine. 2006;31:2151-61.
12. Fardon DF, Milette PC. Nomenclature and classification of lumbar disc pathology. Spine 2001; 26(5):E93-E113.
13. Kang JD, Stefanovic-Racic M, McIntyre LA, Georgescu HI, Evans CH. Toward a biochemical understanding of human intervertebral disc degeneration and herniation: contributions of nitric oxide, interleukins, prostglandin E2, and matrix metalloproteinases. Spine 1997;22:1065-73.
14. Burke JG, Watson RWG, McCormack D, et al. Intervertebral discs which cause low back pain secrete high levels of pro-inflammatory mediators. J Bone Joint Surg (Br). 2002;84-B:196-201.
15. Gilbert HT, Hodson N, Baird P, Richardson SM, Hoyland JA. Acidic pH promotes intervertebral disc degeneration: acid-sensing ion channel -3 as a potential therapeutic target. Sci Rep. 2016;6:37360.

16. Kornman KS. Interleukin 1 genetics, inflammatory mechanisms, and nutrigenetic opportunities to modulate diseases of aging. Am J Clin Nutr. 2006;83(suppl):475S-83S.

17 Diatchenko L, Nackley AG, Slade GD, Fillingim RB, Maixner W. Idiopathic pain disorders - pathways of vulnerability. Pain. 2006;123:226-30.

18. Diatchenko L, Slade GD, Nackley AG et al. Genetic basis for individual variations in pain perception and the development of a chronic pain condition. Human Mol Gen 2005;14:135-43.

19. Edwards RR. Individual differences in endogenous pain modulation as a risk factor for chronic pain. Neurology. 2005;65:437-443.

20. Adams M, Bogduk N, Burton K, Dolan P. The biomechanics of back pain. New York: Churchill Livingstone; 2002: p.78.

21. Souza TA. Differential diagnosis and management for the chiropractor: protocols and algorithms. Gaithersburg: Aspen Pub; 2009: p.144.

22. Schmidt R, Schaible H, Mefslinger K et al. Silent and active nociceptors: structure, functions, and clinical implications. In Gebhart et al. eds. Proc 7th World Congress Pain, 1993, Paris, France. IASP Press: Seattle; 1994: p. 213-250.

23. Mense S. Muscle Pain. Philadelphia: Lippincott, Williams & Wilkins; 2001: p.26-30.

24. Teplik JG, Haskin ME. Spontaneous regression of herniated nucleus pulposus. AJNR Am J Neuroradiol 1985;6:331–35.

25. Doita M, Kanatani T, Ozaki T, et al. Influence of macrophage infiltration of herniated disc tissue on the production of matrix metalloproteinases leading to disc resorption. Spine. 2001; 26:1522-27.

26. Reyentovich A, Abdu WA. Multiple, sequential, and spontaneously resolving lumbar intervertebral disc herniations: a case report. Spine. 2002;27:549-53.

27. Autio RA, Karppinen J, Niinimaki J, et al. Determinants of spontaneous resorption of intervertebral disc herniations. Spine. 2006;31:1247-52

28. Jhawar BS, Fuchs CS, Colditz GA, Stampfer MJ: Cardiovascular risk factors for physician-diagnosed lumbar disc herniation. Spine J 2006;6:684–691.

29. Sakellaridis N. The influence of diabetes mellitus on lumbar intervertebral disk herniation. Surg Neurol 2006;66:152–154.

30. Sakellaridis N, Androulis A. Influence of diabetes mellitus on cervical intervertebral disc herniation. Clin Neurol Neurosurg 2008;110:810–812.

31. Liu X, Pan F, Ba Z, Wang S, Wu D. The potential effect of type 2 diabetes mellitus on lumbar disc degeneration: a retrospective single-center study. J Orthopedic Surg Res. 2018;13:52.

32. Berg G, Miksztowicz V, Schreier L. Metalloproteinases in metabolic syndrome. Clin Chim Acta. 2011;412:1731-39.

33. Hopps E, Caimi G. Matrix metalloproteinases in metabolic syndrome. Eur J Int Med. 2012;23:99-104.

34. Derosa G, Maffioli P, D'Angelo A, et al. Effects of long chain omega-3 fatty acids on metalloproteinases and their inhibitors in combined dyslipidemia patients. Expert Opin Pharmacother. 2009;10:1239-47.

35. Li S, Niu G, Dong XN, Liu Z, Song C, Leng H. Vitamin D inhibits activities of metalloproteinase-9/-13 in articular cartilage in vivo and in vitro. J Nutr Sci Vitaminol. 2019;65:107-112.

36. Timms PM, Mannan N, Hitman GA, et al. Circulating MMP9, vitamin D and variation in the TIMP-1 response with VDR genotype: mechanisms for inflammatory damage in chronic disorders? Q J Med. 2002;95:787-96.

37. Kostov K, Halacheva L. Role of magnesium deficiency in promoting atherosclerosis, endothelial dysfunction, and arterial stiffening as risk factors for hypertension. Int J Mol Sci. 2018;19:1724.

38. Henrotin Y, Clutterbuck AL, Allaway D, et al. Biological actions of curcumin on articular chondrocytes. Osteoarthritis Cart. 2010;18:141-49.

39. Ahmed S, Wang N, Lalonde M, et al. Green tea polyphenol epigallocatechin-3-gallate (EGCG) differentially inhibits interleukin-1b-induced expression of matrix metalloproteinases-1 and -13 in human chondrocytes. J Pharmacol Exper Therapeutics. 2004;308:767-73.

40. Li X, Wang X, Hu Z, et al. Possible involvement of the oxLDL/LOX-1 system in the pathogenesis and progression of human intervertebral disc degeneration or herniation. Scientific Reports. 2017;7:7403.

41. Zhang Y, Zhao Y, Wang M, et al. Serum lipid levels are positively correlated with lumbar disc herniation—a retrospective study of 790 chinese patients. Lipid Health Dis. 2016;15:80.

42. Tsai TT, Ho N, Lin YT, et al. Advanced glycation end products in degenerative nucleus pulposus with diabetes. J Orthop res. 2014;32:238-44.

43. Liu CC, Zhang XS, Ruan YT, et al. Accumulation of methylglyoxal increases the advanced glycation end-product levels in DRG and contributes to lumbar disk herniation-induced persistent pain. J Neurophysiol. 2017;118:1321-28.

44. Segar AH, Fairbank JC, Urban J. Leptin and the intervertebral disc: a biochemical link exists between obesity, intervertebral disc degeneration and low back pain—an in vitro study in a bovine model. European Spine J. 2019;28:214-23.

Chapter 18
Osteoporosis: Diet-induced bone rot

For many years, it has been known that osteoporosis is a state of low-grade chronic inflammation of bone (1-4), which means that osteoporosis is a state of diet-induced bone rot that renders bone weak, fragile, and prone to fracture. Over forty million Americans have reduced bone density (5), which means that osteoporotic bone rot is a serious problem. I outlined some of the dietary inflammation factors related to osteoporosis in a scientific article that was published in 2004 (6). This chapter will expand upon the information in that article.

As outlined earlier in this book and in great detail in *The DeFlame Diet* book, omega-6 fatty acid consumption increases the production of pro-inflammatory prostaglandin E2 (PGE2) (7), and refined sugar, flour, and oils increase the production of pro-inflammatory cytokines (IL-1, IL-6, and TNF) (8). It turns out that an excess of PGE2 and the pro-inflammatory cytokines are all catabolic to bone, which means they degrade bone, which leads to bone loss, called osteopenia. This initially occurs without symptoms and there is no radiological or x-ray evidence until there is 30-50% loss of bone, at which time the individual is diagnosed with osteoporosis.

The only symptom we know of that is associated with osteoporosis is pain if a bone fractures. This means that the osteoporosis develops due to silent pro-inflammatory bone rotting, with no signs or symptoms until the condition is overtly manifested by obvious x-ray evidence and/or fracture.

Women have greater osteoporosis risk than men because estrogen in the normal range is anti-inflammatory, and when production reduces during menopause, there is an associated elevation of inflammatory mediators and a related degradation of bone (8). As menopause is an unavoidable process in the life cycle, women should give great care to maintaining proper bone mass before menopause.

Unfortunately, the ongoing myth is that eating dairy and taking calcium is the best preventive approach. Little to no evidence supports this approach, which is based on the notion that, "calcium is the most abundant mineral in the body and because calcium is the most abundant mineral in bone, women should load up on calcium with dairy and supplements." It would be nice if this worked. However, the evidence that it is a failed approach is demonstrated by the fact that millions of women who load up on calcium and dairy are still being put on osteoporosis drugs, such as Fosamax and Boniva, and other medications outlined in the following section.

Official guidelines for treating osteoporosis
The Agency for Healthcare Research and Quality (AHRQ) is part of the US Department of Health and Human Services. The AHRQ guideline for prevention and treatment of osteoporosis was published in 2011 and includes:

- Lifestyle counseling regarding measures to prevent fractures (exercise, smoking cessation, alcohol restriction, dietary counseling, weight, environmental modification to prevent falls, measures to reduce the impact of falls [such as soft hip protector pads])
- Vitamin D and calcium supplementation
- Pharmacologic agents
  - Gonadal hormone (estrogen) therapy (*prevention*)
  - Bisphosphonates (alendronate, risedronate, ibandronate, zoledronic acid)
  - Selective estrogen receptor modulator (SERM) (raloxifene)
  - Calcitonin (calcitonin-salmon nasal spray)
  - Parathyroid hormone 1-34 (teriparatide)
  - Denosumab
- Follow-up bone mineral density testing (with dual x-ray absorptiometry) at a central site after pharmacologic intervention to assess changes in bone mineral density

This approach to treating osteoporosis is consistent with that which is recommended by the American Academy of Family Physicians (9). Notice that several medications can be used to treat osteoporosis, with estrogen and the bisphosphonates being the most commonly prescribed. If you have osteoporosis, you can expect this approach to be applied to you.

If you do not yet have osteoporosis, my suggestion is that you prevent it from developing by adopting a DeFlaming lifestyle. If you do have osteoporosis and are taking medications, make it your goal to DeFlame your body, which can help to increase your bone density back to normal and free yourself from a reliance on medications.

The lifestyle recommendations in the AHRQ guideline are generally appropriate. The only drawback is that the dietary counseling recommendations, not surprisingly, involve focusing on dairy. Unfortunately, the recommended calcium-supplemented "dairy diet" does not promote bone health because it does not address the cause of osteoporosis, which is chronic inflammation.

The remaining information in this chapter covers the dietary factors that do not make it into official treatment guidelines for osteoporosis. My suggestion would be to eliminate the "dairy diet" in favor of The DeFlame Diet.

Osteoblasts and osteoclasts

More than likely, you have not heard of osteoblasts and osteoclasts, which are the predominant cells found in bone. These are the cells responsible for maintaining normal bone density. The osteoblasts build bone, while the osteoclasts degrade bone. The cells are active throughout life as bone is in a constant state of remodeling or renewing. In other words, the bones you have today are not the same bones you had last year or the years before.

For the remodeling process to be effective and lead to the maintenance of proper bone density, there needs to be a balance in the activity between osteoblasts and osteoclasts. If osteoblast activity is reduced and osteoclast activity is increased, the outcome is bone loss. You need to understand that this imbalance is created by a pro-inflammatory diet and the imbalance cannot be normalized unless the diet is DeFlamed.

Rather than addressing the pro-inflammatory imbalance between osteoclasts and osteoblasts, which is the cause of osteopenia and osteoporosis, a class of drugs called bisphosphonates was developed to inhibit osteoclasts from degrading bone. As indicated in the previous section, there are several bisphosphonates on the market, including Fosamax (alendronate), Boniva (ibandronate), Actonel (risedronate), and Didronel (zoledronic acid).

The problem with bisphosphonates is that osteoclasts are supposed to be active throughout life so they can participate in bone remodeling; they should not be pharmacologically inhibited. It should be understood that the catabolic activity of osteoclasts is supposed to be balanced by osteoblasts that deposit new bone. So to arbitrarily blame osteoclasts for osteoporosis is inappropriate.

Before bisphosphonates were ever tried on humans, we could have predicted that by inhibiting osteoclasts, normal bone remodeling would be disrupted and bone health would decline and perhaps be more prone to damage. In fact, this side effect did emerge with long-term use of bisphosphonates, such that some people developed osteonecrosis of the jaw and fracture of the femur (thigh bone). These side effects are not especially common and so are played down as modern medicine has begun to substantially rely on bisphosphonates to treat osteoporosis. My suggestion is for you to go to drugs.com and search for Fosamax and examine the possible side effects. Identify if these side effects are worth the risk for you.

As with the bisphosphonates and the other medications, supplements cannot restore bone health to rotting osteoporotic bones. DeFlaming the diet is the only way to create the anti-inflammatory body chemistry needed to properly regulate the activities of osteoclasts and osteoblasts.

Multiple dietary inflammation factors participate in bone loss due to the inhibition of bone-building osteoblasts and activation of bone-degrading osteoclasts. When studied individually, these factors may not necessarily appear to be clinically relevant to scientists; however, bone loss becomes clinically relevant when multiple dietary inflammation factors are present in the same person.

Figure 1 lists the multiple dietary inflammation factors that have been identified to promote osteoporotic bone rot. Each factor will be discussed in the remainder of this chapter.

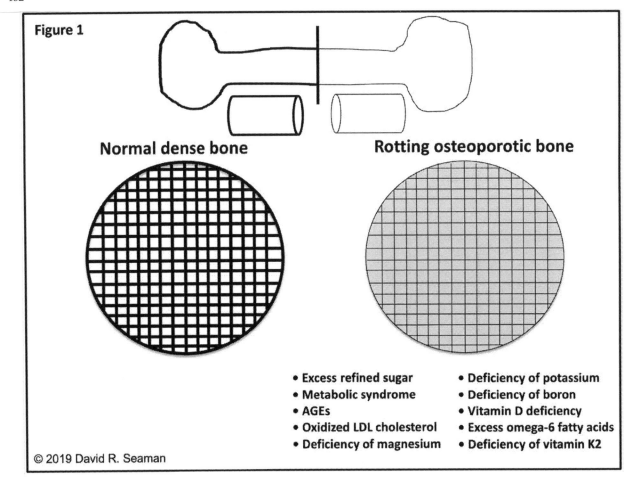

Figure 1

Normal dense bone   Rotting osteoporotic bone

- Excess refined sugar   • Deficiency of potassium
- Metabolic syndrome   • Deficiency of boron
- AGEs   • Vitamin D deficiency
- Oxidized LDL cholesterol   • Excess omega-6 fatty acids
- Deficiency of magnesium   • Deficiency of vitamin K2

© 2019 David R. Seaman

Refined sugar and bone rot

As indicated previously in this book and in all the other DeFlame books, the overconsumption of refined sugar, flour, and oil is the key dietary promoter of chronic inflammation and body rot. As mentioned in Chapter 6, the average American consumes 150 pounds of sugar per year. This amount of sugar has been shown to cause bone loss (10).

When scientists study sugar intake, they use grams rather than ounces or pounds. This means that 150 pounds equates to 67,500 grams of sugar per year, which averages to 185 grams of sugar consumed daily. For perspective, a 20-ounce bottle of Coke contains 65 grams of sugar, so it is not difficult to reach 185 grams each day.

When scientists gave 100 grams of sugar to healthy human subjects, it led to an increase of urinary excretion of key bone minerals, those being calcium, magnesium, and potassium (10). The overconsumption of sugar has additional bone-rotting effects (10):

- Increased osteoclast activity (increased bone degradation)
- Reduced osteoblast activity (reduced bone formation)
- Increased loss of calcium, magnesium, and potassium in the urine

- Decreased intestinal absorption of consumed calcium
- Decreased vitamin D activation

You should realize that refined flour consumption also increases circulating levels of glucose. Consider, for example, a glazed donut from Dunkin Donuts contains 13 grams of refined sugar and another 19 grams of refined flour. So, while there are only 13 grams for pure sugar, there are 32 grams of blood glucose-raising refined carbohydrates.

Metabolic syndrome and osteoporotic bone rot

In the previous section, recall that healthy subjects were fed 100 grams of sugar, which led to a loss of important bone minerals. It should be understood that this effect was only transient because these were healthy subjects. After the hyperglycemic bone-rotting state was over, blood glucose normalized in these subjects and there was no longer a damaging effect delivered to bone. However, when people perpetually overconsume sugar and flour, they will eventually develop the metabolic syndrome or type 2 diabetes. For these people, hyperglycemia is a perpetual state, which means they are living in a perpetual state of body rot that may help to promote osteoporosis (11,12).

Recall from previous chapters that advanced glycation end products (AGEs) accumulate in people with the metabolic syndrome and diabetes and participate in the rotting process of arteries, joints and tendons. The same holds true for bone (13-15). In one study, the authors stated that AGEs could be used to monitor the severity and progression of osteoporosis (15).

Oxidized LDL cholesterol and osteoporotic bone rot

As described in the atherosclerosis chapter (Chapter 13), people with the metabolic syndrome have increased levels of oxidized LDL (oxLDL) cholesterol, which impacts more than just vulnerable arteries. As you read in the joint, tendon, and disc chapters in this book (Chapters 15, 16, & 17), oxLDL participates in the rot that occurs in those tissues. The same holds true for bone.

In 1997, scientists published a study that investigated the reason why atherosclerosis and osteoporosis occur together (16). First, consider this quote from the article:

> "The role of LDL oxidation products and their accumulation in the vessel wall during atherosclerotic lesion formation is well established."

This quote is to emphasize that what I wrote in this book and in *The DeFlame Diet* book about oxidized LDL and atherosclerosis has been considered a scientific fact for many years. It is shameful that the general public is so completely unaware of the difference between regular non-inflammatory LDL and pro-inflammatory oxLDL, which has caused patients to live in fear about cholesterol while they gulp down their statin drugs.

In this 1997 study, the researchers identified that oxLDL has different effects on arteries and bone (16). Oxidized LDL in arteries causes calcium to accumulate in the atherosclerotic plaque. In contrast, oxLDL reduces osteoblast activity, which leads to reduced bone production and reduced calcium accumulation in bone, (16-18), the outcome of which is the bone rot of osteoporosis.

Magnesium deficiency and osteoporotic bone rot

Magnesium deficiency promotes osteoporotic bone rot in several ways. Magnesium deficiency alters the anatomy of a bone component called hydroxyapatite, which leads to reduced bone strength. Magnesium deficiency reduces the activity of osteoblasts and increases osteoclast breakdown of bone. Magnesium deficiency leads to the release of pro-inflammatory cytokines, which also stimulate bone breakdown (5).

Magnesium supplementation in young females and young adult males has led to a reduction in bone turnover (19,20). We are told that, "these findings raise an intriguing possibility that daily oral magnesium supplementation may be used to suppress bone turnover, which subsequently may lead to reduced bone loss and, thus, may have a potential utility for treatment of osteopenia and/or osteoporosis associated with high bone turnover" (20).

In a group of postmenopausal women in Israel suffering from osteoporosis who received magnesium supplements in the range of 250-750 mg/day for 24 months, either bone density increased up to 8% or bone loss was arrested (in 87%); in some cases, both an increase in bone density and arrested bone loss occurred. Untreated controls, on the other hand, lost bone density at an average of 1% a year (21). In another study, a group of postmenopausal osteoporotic women in Czechoslovakia who received magnesium at levels ranging from 1500-3000 mg of magnesium lactate per day for 2 years, nearly 65% were classified totally free of pain and with no further deformity of vertebrae, with the condition in the remainder of the group either arrested or slightly improved (21).

My view, obviously, is that we all need to DeFlame our diets as there is NO magnesium in refined sugar, flour, and oils. I am also an advocate of taking magnesium supplements as described in Chapter 9.

Potassium deficiency and osteoporotic bone rot

While people commonly think that potatoes and bananas are the best source of potassium, in fact, the richest source of potassium is green leafy vegetables. Americans consume precious little green vegetables, which is why most Americans and people in other industrialized nations are potassium deficient. In short, we should be consuming at least 7,000 mg of potassium per day, but most consume about 2500 mg or less (22). This statement is from a review article published in 2001 (22):

> "Increasing potassium intake reduces urinary calcium excretion, which reduces the
> risk of kidney stones and helps prevent bone demineralization."

Experimentally, in the research setting, scientists have supplemented subjects with potassium bicarbonate and potassium citrate, the outcome of which was reduced bone loss (23,24). The best way to increase potassium intake is to eat more fresh fruit and vegetables (22), a topic that is discussed in more detail in the potassium chapter in *The DeFlame Diet* book. Supplemental potassium can lead to cardiac arrhythmias, which is why we should get our potassium from vegetation. Accordingly, a greater consumption of vegetables and fruit is associated with greater bone mineral density (25-27).

Boron deficiency and osteoporotic bone rot

Boron, like magnesium and potassium, has been underappreciated as an important nutrient for bone health. Thus, low boron intake is a relevant nutritional concern, which diets rich in fruits, vegetables, nuts, and legumes can prevent (28). However, the vast majority of individuals do not consume adequate amounts of these natural foods.

The upper limit of boron is set at 20 mg/day (29). The average intake by Americans is approximately 1-3.25 mg/day (28). At the 95th percentile intake, no segment of the US population has a total intake of boron greater than 5 mg/day (29).

Epidemiologic evidence demonstrates that in areas of the world where boron intakes usually are 1.0 mg or less/day, the estimated incidence of arthritis ranges from 20 to 70%, whereas in areas of the world where boron intakes are usually 3 to 10 mg, the estimated incidence of arthritis ranges from 0 to 10%. Bone appears to be stronger in individuals supplemented with boron (30).

Vitamin D deficiency and osteoporotic bone rot

Vitamin D has many different functions as described in Chapter 11. The brief discussion here will be limited to bone health.

First, adequate vitamin D will help to keep cytokine production under control. Without adequate vitamin D, excess cytokines will participate in bone degradation.

Second, vitamin D is needed so the digestive system can absorb calcium. Without adequate vitamin D, calcium absorption will be reduced and lead to lower than normal levels of calcium in the blood. The parathyroid gland responds to low calcium levels by releasing parathyroid hormone. The released parathyroid hormone stimulates osteoclasts to degrade bone and release calcium, which over time, leads to the development of osteoporosis. This scenario, called secondary hyperparathyroidism, can begin to develop when vitamin D levels measured as 25(OH)D fall below 32 ng/ml. In other words, you should find out your 25(OH)D level and get it to at least 70 ng/ml as described in Chapter 11.

Excess dietary omega-6 fatty acids and osteoporotic bone rot

Recall that omega-6 fatty acids are converted into pro-inflammatory prostaglandin E2 (PGE2). It turns out that PGE2 is one of the more potent stimulators of bone degradation and calcium release (31). PGE2 inhibits bone-building osteoblasts and simultaneously stimulates osteoclasts to degrade bone and release calcium (7). Not surprisingly, when there is a proper balance of omega-6 to omega-3 fatty acids, there is a beneficial effect on bone density (32).

Recall from Chapter 2 that we are supposed to have a ratio of omega-6:omega-3 of less than 4 to 1. We can achieve this by eating The DeFlame Diet and taking omega-3 fatty acid supplements. This does require us to eliminate completely, or keep to a bare minimum, the consumption of processed and deep-fried foods that contain refined oils rich in omega-6 fatty acids. The refined oils to eliminate from your diet are from corn, safflower, sunflower, cottonseed, grape seed, peanut, and soybeans.

Gluten and SIBO and osteoporotic bone rot

Celiac disease is the diagnosis given to people who have a strong pro-inflammatory immune reaction to gluten, a protein found in wheat, rye, and barley. The small intestine becomes damaged by chronic inflammation, which is called gluten enteropathy. Gut pain, diarrhea, and bloating are common symptoms. Because the gut wall is damaged, the absorption of nutrients, such as calcium, is impaired, which is called malabsorption. Accordingly, people with celiac disease are more likely to develop osteoporotic bone rot (33,34). Avoiding gluten will restore normal function to the small intestine and improve bone mineral density (34).

SIBO stands for small intestine bacterial overgrowth, which also causes nutrient malabsorption. SIBO develops more commonly in women and is due to a lack of dietary fiber, which is common in the American diet that contains an excess of refined sugar, flour, and oil. SIBO is present in up to 80% of patients with irritable bowel syndrome (IBS) (35). Psychogenic factors also promote IBS (35). No matter the cause, the malabsorption of IBS increases the risk of developing osteoporosis (36,37).

About 1% of the population has celiac disease. Perhaps another 5-10% have gluten sensitivity, which can compromise gut function. When it comes to IBS, it develops in 20% of the US population For more information about each, there are chapters devoted to both gluten and SIBO in *The DeFlame Diet* book.

Vitamin K2 and bone health

In recent years, vitamin K2 has gained notoriety as a nutrient that promotes bone density. You may have come across this information if you try to keep up with nutrition.

There are two types of vitamin K, those being K1 and K2. Phylloquinone (K1) is found in green leafy vegetables. Its primary function is thought to be related to blood clotting. Patients taking warfarin blood thinners, such as Coumadin, function by inhibiting vitamin K. Humans are able to convert vitamin K1 to vitamin K2, however all the details about how this works are not clear. One requirement is eating enough green vegetables, which is rare for most Americans. Fortunately, K2 is also found in food.

Menaquinone is vitamin K2 and there are multiple varieties, which are designated as MK-4 to MK-14. The higher the number, the longer the isoprenoid chain length. You can visualize the differences in chain length by doing an internet search for "vitamin K2 structure." Short chain MK-4 is found in meat. Longer chain MK-7, MK-8, and MK-9 are found in fermented foods such as cheese and curds. MK-7 is also found abundantly in a fermented soybean product called natto. The primary functions of K2 are related to calcium metabolism. Adequate K2 helps to calcify bone and prevent the calcification of arteries.

Vitamin K is interesting because it is known to have only one function. It activates three specific proteins. By activating certain clotting proteins, blood is able to properly clot. By activating blood vessel wall proteins in arteries, the calcification of arteries is prevented. And finally, by activating a bone protein called osteocalcin, proper bone metabolism and bone density are supported.

After identifying that K2 promotes bone density, researchers have supplemented post-menopausal women with 360 mcg of MK-7. The study lasted for a year and bone loss rates were the same for both the supplemented and placebo groups (38). In contrast, another study showed that taking only 180 mcg of MK-7 for three years prevented bone loss in healthy menopausal women (39), suggesting that a longer period of supplementation is required to show a positive effect.

To get adequate K2, we should eat meat, cheese, and eggs. Supplemental K2 is also available in two forms, those being MK-4 and MK-7. I personally use MK-7, as studies have indicated it is the superior form of K2 for artery and bone health. The recommended amount is typically 180 micrograms (mcg) of MK-7.

Summary
After reading this chapter, it should be obvious that multiple factors are involved in preventing our bones from rotting into a state of osteoporosis. By adopting The DeFlame Diet approach to food and supplements, all of these factors are addressed at once.

References
1. Ginaldi L, Di Benedetto MC, De Martinis M. Osteoporosis, inflammation, and ageing. Immun Ageing. 2005;2:14.
2. Mundy GR. Osteoporosis and inflammation. Nutr Rev. 2007;65(12):S147-51.
3. Lacativa PG, de Farias ML. Osteoporosis and inflammation. Arq Bras Endocrinol Metabol. 2010;54(2):123-32.
4. Lencel P, Magne D. Inflammaging: the driving force in osteoporosis? Med Hypoth. 2011;76:317-21.
5. Castiglioni S, Cazzaniga A, Albisetti W, Maier JA. Magnesium and osteoporosis: current state of knowledge and future research directions. Nutrients. 2013;5(8):3022-33.

6. Seaman D. Health care for our bones: a practical nutritional approach to prevent osteoporosis. J Manip Physiol Ther. 2004;27:591-95.

7. Watkins BA, Lippman HE, Le Bouteiller L, et al. Bioactive fatty acids: role in bone biology and bone cell function. Prog Lip Res. 2001;40:125-48.

8. Pfeilschifter J, Koditz R, Pfohl M, Schatz H. Changes in proinflammatory cytokine activity after menopause. Endocrine Reviews. 2002;23(1):90-119.

9. Jeremiah MP, Unwin BK, Greenawald MH, Casano VE. Diagnosis and management of osteoporosis. Am Fam Phys. 2015;92:261-70.

10. DiNicolantonio JJ, Mehta V, Zaman SB, O'Keefe JH. Not salt but sugar as aetiological in osteoporosis: a review. Mo Med. 2018;115:247-52.

11. Yaturu S, Humphrey S, Landry C, Jain SK. Decreased bone mineral density in men with metabolic syndrome alone and with type 2 diabetes. 2009;15(1):CR5-CR9.

12. Yu CY, Chen FP, Chen LW, Kuo SF, Chien RN. Association between metabolic syndrome and bone fracture risk: a community-based study using a fracture risk assessment tool. Medicine. 2017;96(50):e9180.

13. Hein GE. Glycation endproducts in osteoporosis—is there a pathophysiologic importance? Clin Chim Acta. 2006;371:32-36.

14. Yamamoto M, Sugimoto T. Advanced glycation end products, diabetes, and bone strength. Curr Osteoporos Rep. 2016;14:320-26.

15. Yang DH, Chiang TI, Chang IC, et al. Increased levels of circulating advanced glycation end-products in menopausal women with osteoporosis. Int J Med Sci. 2014;453-60.

16. Parhami F, Morrow AD, Balucan J, et al. Lipid oxidation products have opposite effects on calcifying vascular cell and bone cell differentiation. A possible explanation for the paradox of arterial calcification in osteoporotic patients. Arterioscler Thromb Vasc Biol. 1997;17:680-87.

17. Maziere C, Savitsky V, Glamiche A, et al. Oxidized low density lipoprotein inhibits phosphate-induced mineralization in osteoblasts. Involvement of oxidative stress. Biochimica et Biophysica Acta. 2010;1802:1013-19.

18. Maziere C, Salle V, Gomila C, Maziere JC. Oxidized low density lipoprotein enhanced RANKL expression in human osteoblast-like cells. Involvement of ERK, NFkappaB and NFAT. Biochimica et Biophysica Acta. 2013;1832:1756-64.

19. Carpenter TO, DeLucia MC, Zhang JH et al. A randomized controlled study of effects of dietary magnesium oxide supplementation on bone mineral content in healthy girls. J Clin Endocrinol Metab. 2006;91:4866-72.

20. Dimai H-P, Porta S, Wirnsberger G et al. Daily oral magnesium supplementation suppresses bone turnover in young adult males. J Clin Endocrinol Metab. 1998;83:2742-48.

21. Dreosti IE. Magnesium status and health. Nutr Rev 1995; 53(9):S23-S27

22. He FJ, MacGregor GA. Fortnightly review: beneficial effects of potassium. Brit Med J. 2001;323:497-501.

23. Sebastian A, Harris ST, Ottaway JH, Todd KM, Morris RC Jr. Improved mineral balance and skeletal metabolism in postmenopausal women treated with potassium bicarbonate. New Eng J Med. 1994; 330:1776-81

24. Jehle S, Hulter HN, Krapf R. Effect of potassium citrate on bone density, microarchitecture, and fracture risk in healthy older adults without osteoporosis: a randomized controlled trial. J Clin Endocrinol Metab. 2013;98:207-17.

25. Tucker KL, Hannan MT, Chen H, et al. Potassium, magnesium, and fruit and vegetable intakes are associated with greater bone mineral density in elderly men and women. Am J Clin Nutr 1999; 69:727-36

26. New SA, Robins SP, Campbell MK, et al. Dietary influences on bone mass and bone metabolism: further evidence of a positive link between fruit and vegetable consumption and bone health? Am J Clin Nutr. 2000; 71: 142-51

27. Qiu R, Cao WT, Tian HY, et al. Greater intake of fruit and vegetables is associated with greater bone mineral density and lower osteoporosis risk in middle-aged and elderly adults. PLoS One. 2017;12(1):e0168906.

28. Nielsen FH. Is boron nutritionally relevant? Nutr Rev. 2008; 66(4):183-91.

29. National Academy of Sciences. Institute of Medicine. Food and Nutrition Board. Dietary Reference Intakes for Vitamin A, Vitamin K, Arsenic, Boron, Chromium, Copper, Iodine, Iron, Manganese, Molybdenum, Nickel, Silicon, Vanadium, and Zinc. 2001: p.510-521.

30. Newnham RE. Essentiality of boron for healthy bones and joints. Environ Health Perspect. 1994;102(Suppl 7):83-85.

31. Watkins BA, Li Y, Lippman HE, Seifert MF. Omega-3 polyunsaturated fatty acids and skeletal health. Exp Biol Med. 2001; 226:485-97

32. Lavado-Garcia J, Roncero-Martin R, Moran JM, et al. Long-chain omega-3 polyunsaturated fatty acid dietary intake is positively associated with bone mineral density in normal and osteopenic Spanish women. PLoS One. 2018;13(1):e0190539.

33. Capriles VD, Martini LA, Areas JA. Metabolic osteopathy in celiac disease: importance of a gluten-free diet. Nutr Rev. 2009;67:599-606.

34. Larussa T, Suraci E, Imeneo M, et al. Normal bone mineral density associates with duodenal mucosa healing in adult patients with celiac disease on a gluten-free diet. Nutrients. 2017;9:98.

35. Ghoshal UC, Shukla R, Ghoshal U. Small intestinal bacterial overgrowth and irritable bowel syndrome: a bridge between functional organic dichotomy. Gut Liver. 2017;11:196-208.

36. Stobaugh DJ, Deepak P, Ehrenpreis ED. Increased risk of osteoporosis-related fractures in patients with irritable bowel syndrome. Osteoporosis Int. 2013;24:1169-75. (don't have paper)

37. Lee HS, Chen CY, Huang WT, Chang LJ, Chen SC, Yang HY. Risk of fractures at different anatomic cites in patients with irritable bowel syndrome: a nationwide population-based cohort study. Arch Osteoporos. 2018;13:80.

38. Emaus N, Gjesdal CG, Almas B, et al. Vitamin K2 supplementation does not influence bone loss in early menopausal women: a randomized double-blind placebo-controlled trial. Osteoporos Int. 2010;21:1731-40.

39. Knapen MH, Drummen NE, Smit E, Vermeer C, Theuwissen E. Three-year low-dose menaquinone-7 supplementation helps decrease bone loss in healthy postmenopausal women. Osteoporos Int. 2013;24:2499-507.

Chapter 19
Chronic pain and depression: Diet-induced rotting of the nervous system

Chapter 2 introduced various diet-induced pro-inflammatory chemicals that cause the body to rot. Subsequent chapters demonstrated that multiple conditions have these chemicals in common, which means that the dietary and supplementation approach should be essentially the same no matter the condition, including depression. In this Chapter I will explain how it is that chronic pain and depression represent states of chronic diet-induced body rot chemistry.

Chronic pain

The following image was also used as Figure 8 in the disc chapter. The only difference between the two pictures is that the one below says Figure 1 instead of Figure 8.

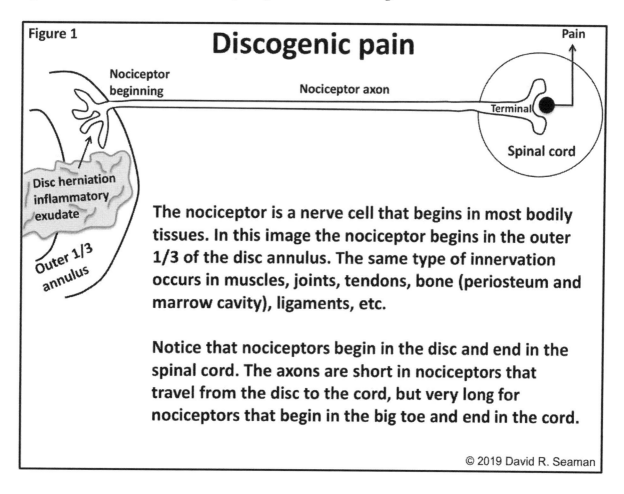

We will use Figure 1 as the introduction to our explanation of pain in this chapter. Recall from the disc chapter that most body tissues are innervated by nerve cells called nociceptors. A key nociceptor function is to sense inflammatory chemistry and once a critical inflammation threshold is reached, the axons transmit inflammation signals to the spinal cord and then to the brain where pain is experienced. As long as the key level of inflammation chemistry persists, pain will also persist.

Figure 1 illustrates nociceptor activation in the disc, which is why the title of the figure is Discogenic Pain. In contrast, the title of Figure 2 is Nociceptive Pain. The image is essentially identical except "disc herniation inflammatory exudate" is replaced by "inflammatory chemistry." You should understand that the nociceptor beginning can start in almost every body tissue and organ. This means that no matter where a pain is, the same chemistry and neurological process is involved.

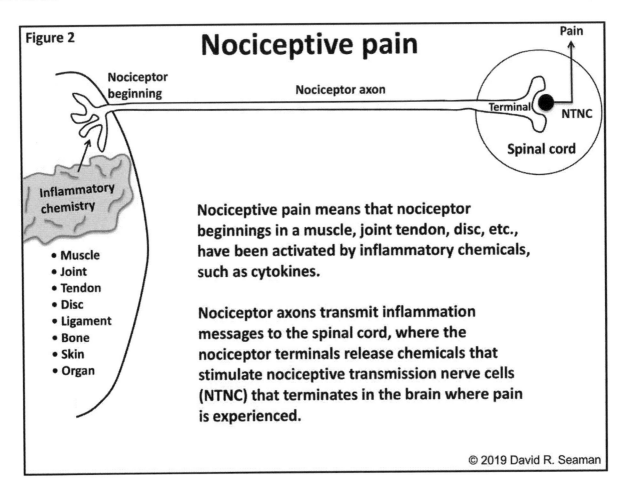

Consider the following pain example. Imagine you are walking across a field and you step in a small hole and roll your ankle over a little so that it hurts. Initially you cannot tell how bad it is, so you stand there and gradually let your body weight distribute onto the leg of the sprained ankle. It does not hurt very much, so you try walking and it turns out that the pain goes away very quickly. In other words, the initial pain was a warning sign of impending damage, NOT actual damage, so a minimal amount of inflammatory chemistry was released rather than a lot. And so, you are able to continue walking across the field without any trouble.

Even if the sprain was a little more severe, with proper rest, it should heal without any additional consequences. Human body physiology includes a healing process that works very efficiently, so long as our lifestyles are not pro-inflammatory. As you learned in this book, when our diets are pro-inflammatory, the outcome is an increased production of inflammatory chemicals. As the "flaming" up process emerges and becomes established as with obesity and vitamin D deficiency, and is regularly augmented by overeating refined sugar, flour, and oil, a pro-inflammatory state of "rot chemistry" is established that prevents effective healing and perpetuates painful symptoms. Figure 3 illustrates how this works at the nociceptor beginning in any tissue that hurts.

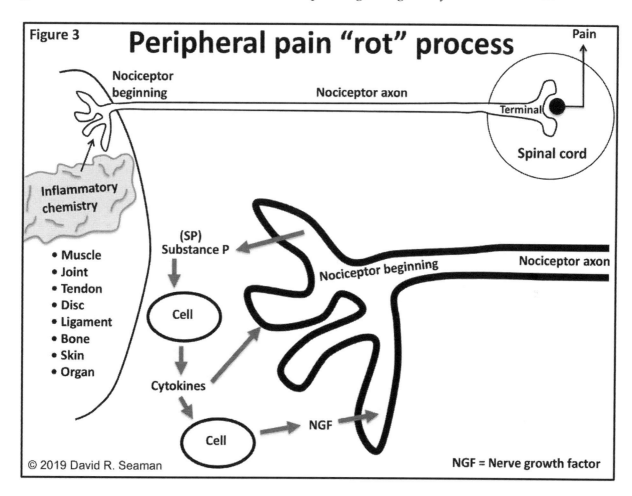

Figure 3

Peripheral pain "rot" process

Pain

Nociceptor beginning

Nociceptor axon

Terminal

Spinal cord

Inflammatory chemistry

- Muscle
- Joint
- Tendon
- Disc
- Ligament
- Bone
- Skin
- Organ

(SP) Substance P

Cell

Nociceptor beginning

Nociceptor axon

Cytokines

Cell

NGF

© 2019 David R. Seaman

NGF = Nerve growth factor

The cells in Figure 3 can be immune cells or fibroblasts, which are common to all tissues. These cells can release a host of inflammatory chemicals; however in Figure 3 only cytokines are illustrated as being released to keep the image less complicated looking.

Cytokines and other inflammatory chemicals bind to their receptor sites on the nociceptor beginning, which causes impulses to be generated in the nociceptor axon, which get transmitted to the spinal cord. Nociceptors not only transmit inflammation signals to the spinal cord, once activated by inflammatory chemicals like cytokines, the nociceptor beginning starts to release a chemical called substance P (SP). After substance P is released, it will stimulate local cells to keep releasing their cytokines and other inflammatory chemicals. The substance P released by nociceptor beginnings is also a key driver in the development of fibrotic or rotting changes in the tissue (1).

> For people with chronic pain, this nociceptor-immune cell-fibroblast cycle of substance P and cytokine release does NOT cease and represents a chronic "peripheral pain rot process."

Tissue cells can also begin releasing nerve growth factor (NGF), which is then taken up by the nociceptor and transported toward the spinal cord. This will happen as long as peripheral inflammation persists. Once NGF travels up the nociceptor and gets near the spinal cord, it functions to dramatically enhance the communication between the nociceptor ending and the nociceptive transmission nerve cell (NTNC) that stimulates the brain to experience pain (2-5).

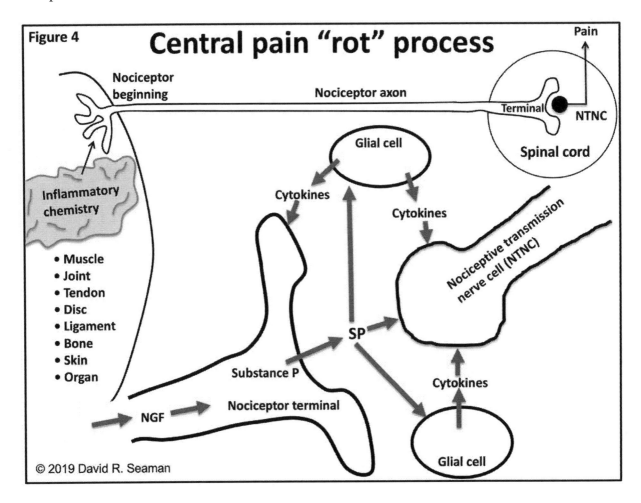

Figure 4 illustrates the central pain "rot" process that will be perpetually active so long as body inflammation persists. Notice that substance P is released by the nociceptor terminal in the spinal cord. Substance P will stimulate the nociceptive transmission nerve cell, also called a spinothalamic tract neuron, which travels from the spinal cord to the brain to create the symptom of pain. Notice that glial cells in the spinal cord are also stimulated by substance P and in response, these glial cells release pro-inflammatory cytokines that stimulate the nociceptor terminal and nociceptive transmission nerve cell (NTNC) to be perpetually stimulated.

> For people with chronic pain, this nociceptor-glial cell-NTNC cycle of substance P and cytokine release does NOT cease and represents a chronic "central pain rot process."

In short, people with chronic pain need to understand that their nervous system's pain communication pathway is perpetually activated by a state of pro-inflammatory body rot chemistry. You could also state it in another way: that the pain pathway is chronically "flamed up" and is readily stimulated to cause pain by activities that should NOT be painful. Scientists refer to this as a sensitized or hyperexcitable pain system, which is always associated with chronic pain.

For some people, taking anti-inflammatory drugs like aspirin and Advil can take the edge off of the pain, but then after the drugs wear off, the pain is back to where it was before the drug was taken. This is a sure sign that the body is chronically flaming and needs to be DeFlamed.

The diet and supplement recommendations in this book have reversed chronic pain for thousands of people who are now living normal, happy lives with minimal to no pain at all. And when these now DeFlamed people get injured, they heal quickly and without disability and pain. The same approach can be applied to depression, which is a pro-inflammatory state of mental and emotional rotting.

Depression
Depression commonly accompanies chronic pain. When both are present, patients often feel especially helpless and hopeless.

In 2011, a report by the World Health Organization (WHO) stated that, "current predictions indicate that by 2030, depression will be the leading cause of disease burden globally" (6). This means that depression is projected to compromise society more than any other condition.

In 2018, another report from the WHO stated that, "depression is the leading cause of disability worldwide, and is a major contributor to the overall global burden of disease" (7). In other words, the 2011 prediction appears to be on track – by 2018 depression was the leading cause of disability, bypassing chronic pain, and by 2030 it will likely be the number one condition that compromises humanity. So, if you have depression and feel alone with your suffering, you should realize that you are not alone by a long shot.

Even if one is young and fit, and lives a healthy lifestyle with an exceptionally DeFlamed diet, it is possible to be thrust into a state of deep depression and despair. The best example of this are certain drone pilots living in America, who develop post-traumatic stress disorder (PTSD) just like combat vets, but these drone pilots NEVER set a boot on the ground in a war zone. In June of 2018, *The New York Times* published an article about this issue entitled: The Wounds of a Drone Warrior (8). So, what happens in the brains of these unfortunate individuals? In short, it has to do with how individual people are not able to tolerate certain mental/emotional stressors.

Everyone has felt stressed more than once in their lives. In fact, most people will say they kind of feel stressed most of the time. Fortunately, most of these people do not develop PTSD or depression, but some do. It turns out that certain stressful thought patterns, based on the individual person's psychology, have the ability to cause glial cells in the brain to chronically release an excess of pro-inflammatory cytokines, which create depression chemistry. This is a bit difficult to conceptualize because this means that thoughts have the ability to stimulate inflammation. Fortunately, scientists have worked out some of the mechanisms.

Cells, including glial cells in the brain, contain a signaling chemical, referred to as an "alarmin" that responds to mental/emotional stressors (9,10). Activation of the alarmin causes glial cells to release pro-inflammatory cytokines (9,10). When this happens chronically, the excess cytokines disrupt normal serotonin and dopamine physiology in brain neurons (nerve cells). Less serotonin and dopamine are produced by nerve cells, less of the produced serotonin and dopamine are released, and each is more rapidly taken up or removed so they cannot be utilized (10,11). Less serotonin makes people feel depressed and act like they are sick. Less dopamine means that the biochemical drive to pursue goals is reduced to a point that people feel no motivation to get through life, to achieve goals, or to pursue fun activities.

It is important for you to know that sedentary living and sleep loss act in the same fashion as mental/emotional stressors to activate the alarmin system. In other words, sedentary living and a lack of sleep create inflammation (12,13), which can become chronic and lead to pain and depression. This relationship has been especially well studied in the context of sleep loss (14,15).

What about diet and depression? You already know that a diet rich in refined sugar, flour, and oil creates chronic inflammation and promotes heart disease, metabolic syndrome, osteoporosis, and painful symptoms in muscles, joints, tendons, and spinal discs. Not surprisingly, the same pro-inflammatory diet promotes depression (16-19). One of the studies demonstrated that overeating fast foods, which are rich in refined sugar, flour, and refined oil, was a predictor for people developing depression after five years (16). The challenge for refined calories eaters is that this cause-effect relationship is blurred because of the five year time span, so these people do not make the connection that their diet caused their depression.

Figure 5 illustrates that the biological rot created by a pro-inflammatory lifestyle leads to depression. It should be obvious that when pain and depression are promoted by a pro-inflammatory diet, a loss of sleep, sedentary living, and poor stress management, there is no way that a meaningful improvement can occur by taking medications. Lifestyle changes are required, and in many cases, they need NOT be exceptionally dramatic. All that one needs to do is improve their lifestyle to the point that the easily measured inflammatory-related markers discussed in Chapter 3 return to normal.

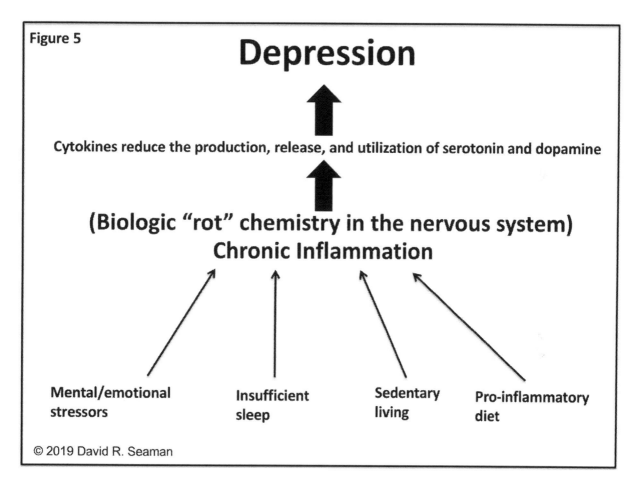

Figure 5

Depression

Cytokines reduce the production, release, and utilization of serotonin and dopamine

(Biologic "rot" chemistry in the nervous system) Chronic Inflammation

Mental/emotional stressors   **Insufficient sleep**   **Sedentary living**   **Pro-inflammatory diet**

© 2019 David R. Seaman

It is important to realize that we essentially have a strong degree of control over our sleep, physical activity level, and our diet. We do not have control over the unforeseen mental/emotional stressors that will impact us, such as death of a loved one, job loss, divorce, personal injury, financial struggles, etc. These mental/emotional stressors can push us over the inflammatory cliff and quickly land us in a state of depression. I have seen this happen to far too many people. We need to fortify our bodies so that we are resilient to such stressors.

If we pursue a pro-inflammatory lifestyle (diet, lack of sleep, sedentary living), we are at risk of turning on the biologic "rot" chemistry of chronic inflammation and launch ourselves into a state of chronic pain and depression while we wait for heart disease, cancer, Alzheimer's disease, etc., to end our lives while loved ones around us suffer. The straightforward information in this book and

168

in *The DeFlame Diet* book can easily address the dietary drive to chronic inflammation and set you free from a great deal of unnecessary suffering.

References

1. Barbe MF, Hilliard BA, Fisher PW, et al. Blocking substance P signaling reduces musculotendinous and dermal fibrosis and sensorimotor declines in a rat model of overuse injury. Connect Tissue Res. 2019;Aug 23:1-16.
2. McMahon SB. NGF as a mediator of inflammatory pain. Phil Trans Royal Soc Lond B. 1996;351:431-40.
3. Woolf CJ. Phenotypic modification of primary sensory neurons: the role of nerve growth factor in the production of persistent pain. Philos Trans R Soc Lond B Biol Sci. 1996; 351(1338):441-48.
4. Woolf CJ, Costigan M. Transcriptional and posttranslational plasticity and the generation of inflammatory pain. Proc Natl Acad Sci. 1999; 96(14):7723-7730.
5. Pezet S, McMahon SB. Neurotrophins: mediators and modulators of pain. Annu Rev Neurosci. 2006; 29:507-38.
6. World Health Organization. December 1, 2011. EB130/9. Executive Board. 130th Session. Global burden of mental disorders and the need for a comprehensive, coordinated response from health and social sectors at the country level.
7. WHO report. March 2018. https://www.who.int/news-room/fact-sheets/detail/depression
8. NY Times. The wounds of a drone warrior. https://www.nytimes.com/2018/06/13/magazine/veterans-ptsd-drone-warrior-wounds.html
9. Frank MG, Weber MD, Watkins LR, Maier SF. Stress sounds the alarmin: the role of danger-associated molecular pattern HMGB1 in stress-induced neuroinflammatory priming. Brain Behav Immun. 2015;48:1-7.
10. Fleshner M, Frank M, Maier SF. Danger signals and inflammasomes: stress-evoked sterile inflammation in mood disorders. Neuropsychopharmacology. 2017;42:36-45.
11. Treadway MT, Cooper JA, Miller AH. Can't or won't? Immunometabolic constraints on dopaminergic drive. Trends Cogn Sci. 2019;23:435-446.
12. de Paula Martins R, Lim CK, Ghisoni K, et al. Treating depression with exercise: the inflammasome inhibition perspective. J Systems Integ Neurosci. 2016;3:1-8.
13. Meier-Ewert HK, Ridker PM, Rifai N, et al. Effect of sleep loss on C-reactive protein, an inflammatory marker of cardiovascular risk. J Am Coll Cardiol. 2004;43:
14. Edwards RR, Almeida DM, Klick B, et al. Duration of sleep contributes to next-day pain report in the general population. Pain. 2008;137:202-207.
15. Al-Abri MA. Sleep deprivation and depression. A bi-directional association. Sultan Qaboos Univ Med J. 2015;15:e4-e6.
16. Akbaraly TN, Brunner EJ, Ferrie JE, et al. Dietary pattern and depressive symptoms in middle age. Brit J Psychiatry. 2009;195:408-13.
17. Crawford GB, Khedkar A, Flaws JA, et al. Depressive symptoms and self-reported fast-food intake in midlife women. Prev Med. 2011;52:254057.
18. Sanchez-Villegas A, Toledo E, Ruiz-Canela M, et al. Fast-food and commercial baked goods consumption and the risk of depression. Public Health Nutr. 2012;15:424-32.
19. Jacka FN, O'Neil A, Opie R, et al. A randomized controlled trial of dietary improvement for adults with major depression (the 'SMILES' trial). BMC Medicine. 2017;15:23.

Chapter 20
Aggressive rotting: Rheumatoid arthritis and other autoimmune diseases

What is an autoimmune disease?
Most people have heard the term autoimmune disease but spend little time thinking about it unless they or family members have one. Rheumatoid arthritis is the most well-known autoimmune disease, but there are many, such as psoriasis, psoriatic arthritis, juvenile rheumatoid arthritis, scleroderma, Sjorgren's syndrome, systemic lupus erythematosus, polymyalgia rheumatica, Hashimoto's disease, multiple sclerosis, and more.

Space does not permit a detailed review of these various autoimmune conditions. The purpose of this chapter is to provide some basic information about autoimmunity, no matter which condition may be present, but the focus will be on rheumatoid arthritis (RA).

The term autoimmunity refers to the process in which the immune system begins to attack tissues of the body. Normally, the immune system responds to foreign proteins called antigens. With autoimmunity, the immune system begins to attack its own body proteins. This shift in immune activity is a gradual process, which is why it takes time for autoimmune diseases to manifest. For example, in the case of rheumatoid arthritis, it typically emerges between the ages of 30-50. This means that time is required for the immune system to substantially flame-up and begin attacking its own body.

About 1 in 100 people have rheumatoid arthritis. The total burden of autoimmune disease is larger, with perhaps about 5% of the world's population being affected (1). People who develop autoimmune diseases are genetically predisposed (2), but that does not mean that expressing the disease is inevitable. In most cases, autoimmune diseases are the outcome of exposing predisposing genes to lifestyle-induced chronic inflammation, which did not exist for humans before the modern day. This is why scientists believe that rheumatoid arthritis, and presumably other autoimmune diseases, may actually be a disease of modern man (3).

Pro-inflammatory dietary choices that drive autoimmunity
The dietary factors that promote autoimmunity are essentially the same as those associated with other chronic conditions of the musculoskeletal system and visceral organs. In other words, the nutritional information in this book and in *The DeFlame Diet* book apply to autoimmunity. In short, most people in America live on a diet that is promotional for autoimmune disease expression.

Chapters earlier in this book clearly outline how obesity and the metabolic syndrome are chronic pro-inflammatory states. Not surprising, both obesity and the metabolic syndrome are known to be promoters of autoimmune disease (4-6). Indeed, "obesity appears to be a major environmental factor contributing to the onset and progression of autoimmune diseases." (4). And, the pro-inflammatory state of the metabolic syndrome, "may participate in the onset and persistence of rheumatoid arthritis" (6). With this in mind, I have never met anyone with rheumatoid arthritis who has been told by their rheumatologist or personal physician to aggressively alter the diet to eliminate obesity and the metabolic syndrome; they are just given medications and told to learn to live with it.

In 1991, an article was published that described 27 patients with RA who stayed at a health farm for 4 weeks, wherein they adopted an entirely different dietary program. After a 7-10 day partial fast, which consisted of herbal teas, garlic, vegetable broth, a decoction of potatoes and parsley, and juice extracts from carrots, beets and celery; each subject was placed on an individually adjusted gluten-free vegan diet for 3-5 months. Within the first 4 weeks, there was a significant improvement in symptoms, which were still present after one year (7). Most of the subjects were counseled to maintain a gluten-free vegan diet or a lactovegetarian diet. The key to understanding the effectiveness of this dietary change is understand that refined sugar, flour, and oils were eliminated. These are the calories that are a creation of modern man. In other words, you can be a vegan, omnivore, or carnivore if you have autoimmune disease. Let your tracking of inflammation markers be your dietary guide.

A lack of anti-inflammatory omega-3 fatty acids in the diet appears to be a promoter of rheumatoid arthritis. A rheumatologist (Dr. Joel Kremer) at Albany Medical College pioneered the use of high dose fish oil supplements in the treatment of rheumatoid arthritis (8,9). His studies involved patients who only took fish oil in addition to whatever medications they were taking. In other words, no dietary changes were made at all. He discovered that at least 3 grams of omega-3 fatty acids, called eicosapentaenoic acid (EPA) and docosahexaenoic acid (DHA), from fish oil need to be taken for at least 12 weeks before a clinical effect may be noticed. Some of the subjects who took 3-6 grams of EPA/DHA had such a positive outcome that they were able to discontinue taking medications (8).

As described earlier in this book, a lack of vitamin D causes the immune system to become pro-inflammatory. The immune cell shift described in Chapter 11 is an autoimmune profile. In the context of this chapter, people do not realize that vitamin D deficiency is pervasive in patients with autoimmune diseases (10). In other words, anyone with rheumatoid arthritis or any other autoimmune disease, needs to have their vitamin D levels checked and maintained at an anti-inflammatory level, which appears to be about 70 ng/ml.

Ginger supplementation was already discussed a bit in Chapter 9. In 1992, scientists published a paper that described various individuals with osteoarthritis or rheumatoid arthritis who ate ginger or used ginger powder (11). The typical amount that people took was 2-6 grams of ginger per day. A 50 year-old male with rheumatoid arthritis ate up to 50 grams per day as part of his cooked vegetable and meat dishes. Relief in pain and swelling was evident after 1 month of ginger intake. He was completely free of pain and swelling after 3 months of ginger consumption. He was active as an automobile mechanic, and 13-14 years passed without relapse of symptoms. Eventually, some rheumatoid nodules appeared on some of the joints of the fingers of both hands without any deformity and loss of function or pain.

In 2000, Dr. Loren Cordain and his colleagues wrote an article that outlined how lectins from grains and legumes may alter gut permeability and allow for the absorption of dietary and bacterial antigens to be absorbed and function as promoters of autoimmunity (12). To inactivate lectins, grains and legumes should be pressure cooked. As a side note, if you like the paleodiet concept, my suggestion is that you follow the work of Dr. Cordain who founded this dietary movement. It was Dr. Cordain who turned me on to the fact that the excessive amount of salt in the modern diet may play a role in promoting autoimmunity (13).

Gluten ingestion can also be a promoter of autoimmunity. For example, celiac disease is an autoimmune disease that is caused by gluten consumption. About 1 in 100 people have celiac disease (14). In the case of rheumatoid arthritis, in 1964, a study was published that involved 18 patients who went gluten free. All 18 patients improved on a gluten-free diet, often within two weeks after beginning the diet (15). Many people get tested for gluten sensitivity or celiac disease, which is fine. However, the easiest and cheapest way to see if gluten is negatively impacting you, is to simply avoid eating gluten and see if your symptoms improve.

Gut health has become especially popular in recent years. Studies have shown that dysbiosis can play a role in the development of rheumatoid arthritis (16). The term dysbiosis is applied to an abnormal gut bacterial population that is most commonly caused by eating a pro-inflammatory diet. For more information, *The DeFlame Diet* book has individual chapters devoted to gluten and small intestine bacterial overgrowth (SIBO) and includes a simple eating test to distinguish between the two conditions.

Infections (17,18) and increased levels of female hormones in men and women (19,20) can participate in autoimmune disease expression. These issues are not typically investigated when patients are treated for autoimmune disease. People with autoimmune diseases should identify if they have a low-grade infection or elevated female hormones. Whether or not there is an infection or female hormone issue, the diet of a person with autoimmunity needs to be drastically DeFlamed.

References

1. Amador-Patarroyo MJ, Rodriguez-Rodriguez A, Montoya-Ortiz G. How does age at onset influence the outcome of autoimmune diseases? Autoimmune Diseases. 2016; Article ID: 251730.
2. Oliver JE, Silman AJ. What epidemiology has told us about risk factors and aetiopathogenesis in rheumatic diseases. Arth Res Ther. 2009;11(3):223.
3. Kavanaugh AF, Lipsky PE. Rheumatoid arthritis. In: Gallin JI, Synderman R. Eds. Inflammation: basic principles and clinical correlates. 2nd ed. Philadelphia: Lippincott Williams & Wilkins; 1999: p.1017-1037.
4. Versini M, Jeandel PY, Rosenthal E, Shoenfeld Y. Obesity and autoimmune diseases: not a passive bystander. Autoimmun Rev. 2014;13:981-1000.

5. Dessein PH, Joffe BI, Stanwix AE. Effects of disease modifying agents and dietary intervention on insulin resistance and dyslipidemia in inflammatory arthritis: a pilot study. Arthritis Res 2002;4(6):R12. Epub.

6. Dessein PH, Stanwix AE, Joffe BI. Cardiovascular risk in rheumatoid arthritis versus osteoarthritis: acute phase response related decreased insulin sensitivity and high-density lipoprotein cholesterol as well as clustering of metabolic syndrome features in rheumatoid arthritis. Arthritis Res. 2002;4(5):R5. Epub.

7. Kjeldsen-Kragh J, Haugen M, Borchgrevink CF et al. Controlled trial of fasting and one-year vegetarian diet in rheumatoid arthritis. Lancet . 1991; 338:899-902.

8. Kremer JM. n-3 fatty acid supplements in rheumatoid arthritis. Am J Clin Nutr 2000;71(1 Suppl):349S-51S.

9. Kremer JM. Fish oil and inflammation – a fresh look. J Rheumatol. 2017;44:713-16.

10. Haroon M, Bond U, Quillinan N, Phelan MJ, Regan MJ. The prevalence of vitamin D deficiency in consecutive new patients seen over a 6-month period in general rheumatology clinics. Clin Rheumatol. 2011;30:789–794.

11. Srivistava KC, Mustafa T. Ginger (Zingiber officinale) in rheumatism and musculoskeletal disorders. Med Hypothesis. 1992;39:342-48.

12. Cordain L, Toohey L, Smith MJ, Hickey MS. Modulation of immune function by dietary lectins in rheumatoid arthritis. Brit J Nutr. 2000;83:207-17.

13. Sigaux J, Semerano L, Favre G, Bessis N, Boissier MC. Salt, inflammatory joint disease, and autoimmunity. Joint Bone Spine. 2018;85:411-16.

14. Casado MA, Lorite P, Ponce de Leon C, Palmeque T. Celiac disease autoimmunity. Arch Immunol Ther Exp. 2018;66:423-30.

15. Shatin R. Preliminary report of the treatment of rheumatoid arthritis with high protein gluten-free diet and supplements. Med J Aust. 1964;2:169-72.

16. Horta-Baas G, Romero-Figueroa M, Montiel-Jarquin AJ, et al. Intestinal dysbiosis and rheumatoid arthritis: a link between gut microbiota and the pathogenesis of rheumatoid arthritis. J Immunol Res. 2017;2017:4835189.

17. Sfriso P, Ghirardello A, Bostsios C, et al. Infections and autoimmunity: the multifaceted relationship. J Leukoc Biol. 2010;87:385-95.

18. Ercolini AM, Miller SD. The role of infections in autoimmune disease. Clin Exper Immunol. 2008;155:1-15.

19. Tengstrand B, Carlstrom K, Fellander-Tsai L, Hafstrom I. Abnormal levels of serum dehydroepiandrosterone, estrone, and estradiol in men with rheumatoid arthritis: high correlation between serum estradiol and current degree of inflammation. J Rheumatol. 2003;30(11):2338-43.

20. Jara LJ, Medina G, Saavedra MA, et al. Prolactin and autoimmunity. Clinic Rev Allerg Immunol. 2011;40:50-59.

Chapter 21
The opioid crisis and our rotting bodies

At this point, there should be no doubt in your mind that the average American is living on a pro-inflammatory diet that is gradually causing their bodies to rot. Without knowing it, this is how people are putting themselves at risk for opioid addiction. Here are some facts to consider:

1. People with rotting, pro-inflammatory bodies are more likely to suffer with pain.
2. The fat mass of obese people releases pro-inflammatory cytokines, which causes obese people to be more likely to suffer with chronic pains.
3. Depressed people commonly suffer with pain, as depression and pain chemistry is essentially identical.

With the above in mind, you should not be surprised that obese people are more likely to become opioid addicts compared to normal weight people (1). The same holds true for depressed people; they are more likely to become opioid addicts (2).

For more information about the opioid crisis, you can download a chapter I co-wrote for one of Jack Canfield's recent books entitled, *The Recipe For Success*. Jack Canfield is most well-known for his book, *Chicken Soup for the Soul*. The title of our chapter is, "A success plan for pain-free living: an antidote for the opioid crisis." The chapter is available on the blog section of DeFlame.com:

https://deflame.com/blog/wp-content/uploads/2018/12/Drs-Rosa-Seaman-2C-Opioid-Chapter-C-Canfield-book2C-2019.pdf

The obvious answer to dealing with chronic inflammation and pain is to DeFlame the diet. This should be married to lifestyle that involves exercise, proper sleep and stress management.

I will likely be writing a book about the opioid crisis with my Canfield chapter co-author and friend, Dr. John Rosa. We will outline the nature of the crisis, the lifestyle factors that drive chronic pain and inflammation, and how to manage chronic pain patients from an integrative medicine perspective. We hope to have this book published sometime in 2020.

References
1. Stokes A, Berry KM, Collins JM, et al. The contribution of obesity to prescription opiod use in the United States. Pain. 2019;160:2255-62.
2. Grattan A, Sulivan MD, Saunders KW, Campbell CI, Von Korff MR. Depression and prescription opioid misuse among chronic opioid therapy recipients with no history of substance abuse. Ann Fam Med. 2012;10:304-11.

Chapter 22
Final thoughts: Embracing the body rot concept

As I stated in the introduction, most people have a misconception about the nature of chronic inflammation. As illustrated by the images in the chapters about obesity, atherosclerosis, muscle rot, osteoarthritis, tendinosis, disc herniation, and osteoporosis, there are actually anatomy changes that occur in these tissues, which take on the appearance of a "biologic rot" process. The rotting is especially intense in people with autoimmune diseases that attack various tissues and organs.

There are obviously many conditions that I did not discuss in this book; however, that should not stop you from applying the body rot concept to essentially any condition. For example, Alzheimer's disease and Parkinson's disease are examples of brain rot conditions. Fatty liver and cirrhosis are liver rot conditions. The term 'gut rot" can apply to many conditions, such as irritable bowel syndrome, ulcerative colitis, and Crohn's disease. All cancers represent biologic rot conditions; they are just typically far more life-threatening compared to rotting joints and tendons, which are just chronically painful. All of these conditions should be combatted by DeFlaming the body.

By embracing the body rot concept, you automatically have to take into consideration all of the dietary issues described in this book, which is not how diseases are viewed by many in the healthcare field. This is especially problematic for medical doctors who choose to only prescribe medications and do not adequately urge patients to change their diets and lifestyles to get their inflammatory markers into the normal range. If I was a medical doctor, I would likely prescribe certain medications based on the diagnosed condition…but this would only be a short-term scenario. My goal would be to normalize the markers of inflammation and eliminate the need for drug prescriptions or drastically minimize the need for drugs.

In contrast with medical doctors, other popular healthcare providers cannot prescribe medications. These include chiropractors, physical therapists, psychologists, massage therapists, and acupuncturists. A challenge for these providers is that the chronically inflamed and rotting population commonly does not respond to their treatments. If these providers DeFlame their non-responding patients, their treatments will be much more successful. The same holds true for dental treatments, with the best example being dental implants.

Dentists know that implants are less effective in obese people with diabetes, which is made worse if these people also smoke. In short, the mouths of obese diabetic smokers are much more likely to be rotting with chronic inflammation, which does not allow for an effective healing process after an implant.

Our healthcare crisis

I briefly discussed the opioid crisis in the previous chapter, which is part of a greater healthcare crisis. The topic of healthcare is a hot-button social and political debate and in my view, the debate misses a key issue. The uninsured and the high expense of healthcare are the typical issues that are talked about. This misses the key issue which is…who is it that needs healthcare?

The lion's share of healthcare spending goes to people with rotting bodies that need drugs and surgery. This means that billions and billions of dollars are spent annually on medications and surgery that would otherwise be unnecessary if multiple millions of Americans were not chronically inflamed and literally rotting. These are the same people who add another layer to healthcare costs, which is related to disability expenditures. Multiple additional billions of dollars are spent on people who were injured and now disabled with chronic pain. Most of these people were rotting before they got injured, which prevented them from healing properly and getting on with their lives.

In short, our healthcare system is in trouble because multiple millions of people with rotting bodies are seeking help who could otherwise help themselves by DeFlaming. These people only need drugs and surgery because they pursued a lifestyle that led them to the point where they need expensive drugs and surgery. I personally have no interest in needing medication or surgery.

Even if drugs and surgeries were free, I would still not want either. Only rotting bodies need these interventions and a rotting body is all about suffering and misery. If I can live the rest of my life without medications and surgery, it will be a good life. That is because life is difficult, painful, and challenging enough without the added misery of a rotting body and mind that needs to be highly medicated and hospitalized.

A great benefit to society would emerge if people DeFlamed their bodies. There would be far less stress placed on our healthcare system, such that money could be made available to help the truly needy who were injured or developed conditions based on an unfortunate collection of pro-inflammatory genes.

The easiest way to begin the DeFlaming process

This is the same section that can be found at the end of Chapter 1. The easiest way to start DeFlaming is reduce the number of hours spent each day eating, which is called time-restricted feeding (TRF). I think it is wise for everyone to fast at least 13 hrs per night and try to extend it to at least 18 hours based on one's individual comfort level, and this is because TRF is anti-inflammatory (1-3). Even if one eats the same pro-inflammatory calories, it is much better to do it in an 6-11 our eating window or less. Consider this real-life example.

I met a guy who told me that at the age 45 he was diagnosed with type 2 diabetes. At the time of the diagnosis his weight was 250 pounds, while his proper weight was 200 pounds. Because he did not want to take medications for the rest of his life, this man decided to eat just 600 calories per day within a 6-hr time period until he got his weight back to 200 lbs. For 3 months he ate a double cheeseburger from MacDonald's, which was about 450 calories. The remaining 150 calories was vegetables and fruit. At the end of the 3 months, he weighed 200 pounds again and no longer had diabetes.

I am not suggesting that anyone should do the double cheeseburger plan. The point of this example is to illustrate that there are many ways to DeFlame. My suggestion is to drastically avoid refined sugar, flour, and oils whether one chooses to be a vegan, omnivore, or carnivore and then let the normalization of inflammatory markers be the ultimate eating guide. In most cases, it is not a requirement for the diet to be ketogenic, so go keto only if it suits your individual preferences. Whichever foods you choose to eat, begin with a 13-hr fast and then extend it based on your comfort level, which vary day to day.

References

1. Marinack CR, Nelson SH, Breen CI, et al. Prolonged nightly fasting and breast cancer prognosis. JAMA Oncol. 2016;2:1049-55.
2. Moro T, Tinsley G, Bianco A, et al. Effects of eight weeks of time-restricted feeding (16/8) on basal metabolism, maximal strength, body composition, inflammation, and cardiovascular risk factors in resistance-trained males. J Translational Med. 2016;14:290.
3. Jamshed H, Beyl RA, Della Manna DL, et al. Early time-restricted feeding improves 24-hour glucose levels and affects markers of the circadian clock, aging, and autophagy in humans. Nutrients. 2019;11:1234.

Index

Printed in Poland
by Amazon Fulfillment
Poland Sp. z o.o., Wrocław